Nathalie Moshfegh

Feeding behavior of laboratory dogs during animal testing

Nathalie Moshfegh

Feeding behavior of laboratory dogs during animal testing

Feeding behavior of laboratory dogs as a helpful guideline to their state of health during animal testing

Südwestdeutscher Verlag für Hochschulschriften

Impressum / Imprint
Bibliografische Information der Deutschen Nationalbibliothek: Die Deutsche Nationalbibliothek verzeichnet diese Publikation in der Deutschen Nationalbibliografie; detaillierte bibliografische Daten sind im Internet über http://dnb.d-nb.de abrufbar.
Alle in diesem Buch genannten Marken und Produktnamen unterliegen warenzeichen-, marken- oder patentrechtlichem Schutz bzw. sind Warenzeichen oder eingetragene Warenzeichen der jeweiligen Inhaber. Die Wiedergabe von Marken, Produktnamen, Gebrauchsnamen, Handelsnamen, Warenbezeichnungen u.s.w. in diesem Werk berechtigt auch ohne besondere Kennzeichnung nicht zu der Annahme, dass solche Namen im Sinne der Warenzeichen- und Markenschutzgesetzgebung als frei zu betrachten wären und daher von jedermann benutzt werden dürften.

Bibliographic information published by the Deutsche Nationalbibliothek: The Deutsche Nationalbibliothek lists this publication in the Deutsche Nationalbibliografie; detailed bibliographic data are available in the Internet at http://dnb.d-nb.de.
Any brand names and product names mentioned in this book are subject to trademark, brand or patent protection and are trademarks or registered trademarks of their respective holders. The use of brand names, product names, common names, trade names, product descriptions etc. even without a particular marking in this works is in no way to be construed to mean that such names may be regarded as unrestricted in respect of trademark and brand protection legislation and could thus be used by anyone.

Coverbild / Cover image: www.ingimage.com

Verlag / Publisher:
Südwestdeutscher Verlag für Hochschulschriften
ist ein Imprint der / is a trademark of
AV Akademikerverlag GmbH & Co. KG
Heinrich-Böcking-Str. 6-8, 66121 Saarbrücken, Deutschland / Germany
Email: info@svh-verlag.de

Herstellung: siehe letzte Seite /
Printed at: see last page
ISBN: 978-3-8381-3682-0

Zugl. / Approved by: Zürich, Universität Zürich, Diss., 2012

Copyright © 2013 AV Akademikerverlag GmbH & Co. KG
Alle Rechte vorbehalten. / All rights reserved. Saarbrücken 2013

Table of Contents

1. Zusammenfassung / Summary 1
2. Introduction 2
   2.1 Feeding system at Novartis 2
   2.2 Definition of "wellbeing" 3
      2.2.1 Physiological and behavioral indicators of wellbeing 3
      2.2.2 Pain 4
      2.2.3 Suffering 4
      2.2.4 Injury 5
      2.2.5 Anxiety 5
      2.2.6 Stress 5
   2.3 Physiological measure of stress and distress 6
   2.4 Severity grade of the constraint of the dog 7
      2.4.1 No distress: Severity Grade 0 7
      2.4.2 Minor distress: Severity Grade 1 7
      2.4.3 Moderate distress: Severity Grade 2 7
      2.4.4 Severe distress: Severity Grade 3 7
3. General behavior of dogs 8
   3.1. Behavioral signals 8
   3.2 Feeding behavior of dogs: General facts 8
      3.2.1 Palatability of the food: taste texture, and smell 9
   3.3 Control of the digestion and food intake 9
      3.3.1 Central mechanism 10
      3.3.2 Hunger, satiety and satiation 10
      3.3.3 Gastrointestinal control 10
      3.3.4 Metabolic and neurochemical Influence on satiety 11
      3.3.5 Polyphagia and Anorexia 11
      3.3.6 Taste Aversion 12
   3.4 Drug discovery and development process – an Overview 12
      3.4.1 Target discovery 12
      3.4.2 Drug discovery 13

3.4.3 Safety and drug metabolism	13
3.4.4 Clinical trial I-II	14
3.4.5 Clinical trial III	14
3.4.6 Registration and Pharmacovigilance	14
3.5 Different kind of studies in toxicology	14
3.5.1 Compound selection studies	14
3.5.2 Dose selection studies	14
3.5.3 Regulatory studies	14
3.6 Aim of this study	15
4. Materials und Methods	16
4.1 Animals	16
4.1.1 Procedure from the first entry of dogs to the end of the study	16
4.2 Housing facilities	16
4.3 Study data material	18
4.4 Structure of a regulatory-study	19
4.4.1 Pretest	19
4.4.2 Main phase = treatment phase	19
4.4.3 Recovery	20
4.5 In-life examinations	20
4.5.1 Clinical observations	20
4.5.2 Body weight	20
4.5.3 Food consumption	20
4.5.4 ECG	21
4.5.5 Ophthalmology	21
4.5.6 Neurology	21
4.5.7 Clinical pathology: hematology, clinical biochemistry and urinalysis	21
4.5.9 Toxicokinetics and special investigation	22
4.5.10 Pathology	22
4.6 Dog feeding system	22
4.6.1 Dog feeder	22
4.6.2 Implant	24

4.6.3 Situations that may occur during the feeding process 25

4.6.4 Display and control units 25

4.6.5 Meal Definition 26

4.6.6 Use and function of FeeditManager 27

4.6.7 Errors occurring during feeding process 29

4.7 Statistical Evaluation 30

5. Results 31

5.1 General food intake behavior 31

5.1.1 Body weight 39

5.2. Three feeding patterns and their examples 39

5.2.1 First example: Study A with no Impact 40

5.2.2 Second example: Study B with irregular impact 43

5.2.3 Third example: Study C with a clear impact at the beginning of the dosing part of both sexes 50

5.2.4 Fourth example: Study D with a clear impact, not only in high dose groups 53

5.2.5 Fifth example: Study E with an increasing food consumption 58

5.4 Total visits 64

5.5. Symptoms 65

6. Discussion 68

6.1 Thoughts regarding group housing dogs 68

6.2 Observations of daily food intake in the pretest, main phase, and the recovery phase 70

6.2.1 Pretest 71

6.2.2 Main phase 72

6.2.3 Recovery 73

6.2.4 Single meals 74

6.2.5 DFI and visits 75

6.2.6 DFI and MDT 75

6.2.7 DFI and symptoms 75

6.2.8 Feeding behavior and pathological findings 76

6.2.9 Correlation between food intake and clinical parameters 76

6.3 Conclusion 76

7. References 78
8. Abbreviations 85
9. Appendix 87

1. Zusammenfassung / Summary

Die Analyse des Futterkonsums zur Beurteilung des Gesundheitszustandes der Tiere, vor allem bei Ratten, ist ein weit verbreiteter Indikator in verschiedenen Gebieten.
Das Fressverhalten von Versuchshunden ist nur wenig beschrieben und es gibt kaum publizierte Literatur darüber.

Novartis PCS Toxikologie Schweiz verwendet Futterautomaten zur genaueren Messung des Futterkonsums der Versuchshunde.

Das Ziel dieser Studie war es, das normale Fressverhalten von Versuchshunden während der Pretest-Phase zu definieren und ein Fressprofil zum Vergleich mit der Hauptversuchsphase zu erstellen.
Es wurden Beobachtungen gemacht, welche eine Veränderung der Fressprofile aufdeckten und somit eine hilfreiche Richtlinie zur Beurteilung des Gesundheitszustandes der Hunde darstellten.
Anhand der Daten von sechzehn Toxikologie Studien mit oraler Applikation der letzten drei Jahre wurde eine Definition für die Mahlzeit erstellt. Die Studien bestanden aus einer zwei bis vier Wochen Versuchsphase mit einer vier-wöchigen Erholungsphase. Die Fressprofile der Hunde der verschiedenen Studienphasen wurden miteinander verglichen. Auch die Fressprofile der verschiedenen Dosisgruppen mit den Kontrollgruppen wurden verglichen. Es wurden Abweichungen vom normalen Fressverhalten beobachtet, vor allem in der Gruppe mit der höchsten Dosis, manchmal aber auch in Gruppen der tieferen Dosis.
Anhand der Resultate kann gesagt werden, dass das Fressverhalten ein wichtiger und sensitiver Indikator zur Beurteilung des Wohlbefindens der Versuchshunde ist.

The collection and analysis of food consumption data is widely used as a parameter to monitor the health status of animals, especially in rats, in a variety of areas.
However, the feeding behavior in laboratory dogs has not been described in detail and there is only little literature available in the public domain.

Novartis PCS Toxicology Switzerland is using automated feeding machines to record the food consumption of individual dogs.

The aim of this study was to determine the normal feeding behavior of untreated laboratory dogs during the pretest period and to create a feeding profile for comparison with the main study phase.
Observations were made that identified any modified patterns of feeding behavior, which can be a helpful guideline for the dogs' state of wellness, especially if no other symptoms are present.
On the basis of data from 459 dogs the definition of a single meal intake was established. Sixteen two to four-week oral toxicity studies with a four-week recovery period over the last three years were analyzed. A comparison of the feeding pattern was made during the pretest, the main study and the recovery period for each dog.
Feeding profiles between the different dosing groups compared with the control group were also analyzed.
In general, deviations were seen from the normal feeding pattern, especially in the high dose group and sometimes even in lower dose groups regardless of the presentation of other clinical symptoms.
Overall, the results of this study show, that the feeding behavior of dogs is a helpful and sensitive tool to evaluate the health status of laboratory dogs.

2. Introduction
Food consumption is one of the most sensitive parameters for the general health and wellbeing of both animals and man.

It is quite common to analyze feeding behavior and food consumption in rats with automated "eatometers" to study physiological control of feeding. These options are also used for obesity research to evaluate the efficacy and specificity of agents that stimulate or inhibit feeding (HULSEY MARTIN G et al 1991), especially in combination with metabolic diseases.

Another interesting use of automated feeding systems can be seen in farming. Feed is a major cost of domestic livestock and to optimize the cost to meat ratio it is very helpful to know heritability of food intake as well as correlations between food intake and other parameters of economic importance (CAMMACK et al 2005).
For example, investigations in farming were made to study stressors on swine growth (Y. Hyun et al.), to control the health status of weaning pigs (BRUININX et al 2001) or to investigate effects of probiotic administration in swine (ROSS et al 2010)

MADRID et al (1993) described various methods to record the feeding behavior of rats
- Operant methods: the animal has to press a bar to get food
- Pellet-detecting eatometer deliver a pellet each time, the first one is eaten
- Electronic balances measure the food and send the information to a computer
- Devices which record the presence of the whole animal or the animal's head.
- Devices which detect the animal's contact with the food (eatometers)

Only a small number of studies or papers about feeding behavior of laboratory dogs or implemented feeding machines for dogs used for animal testing have been published (RASHOTTE et al 1988, BRADSHAW 1991).

A large number of animals over a long time period are necessary to make the records usable (MADRID et al 1993). The high costs and the time-consuming work up of the data are probably the main reason why this has not yet been established for dogs.

2.1 Feeding system at Novartis
Before Novartis Pharma AG (Division NIBR, Preclinical safety, Toxicology, building 126.1, Klybeck, Basel, Switzerland) implemented their self invented automated feeding machines in cooperation with *Itin&Hoch, Liestal* (Hardware) and *Christian Waldmann (RealTime Engineering), Gelterkinden* (Software) experimental dogs were fed manually. The dogs were separated for at least 3 hours for feeding time and the residuals of the meal were weighed back and recorded in the program. By limiting the time to feed, only limited individual variability in food consumption was possible.
This manual feeding had the following disadvantages:

- Animals had to be separated to feed
- Animals had only 3-4 hours time to eat, which differs from their normal feeding behavior, when fed *ad libitum*
- Only limited information about the feeding patterns was available (even though the food consumption is an important parameter, especially for toxicology studies)
- As dogs were fed *ad libitum* at the breeding station outside Novartis, animals were not used to be fed over a limited time period and therefore an extended acclimatization period was required.
- Animal welfare constraints: Animals should be kept separated on a minimum of time
- Manually feeding is more time consuming than using an automated feeding system

- Only limited distinction between lower food intake related to the study and lower food intake due to limited access to food is possible

With the new way of feeding, the dogs did not have to be separated anymore. They could live out their natural feeding behavior and it was also possible, to record the individual visits, the amount eaten during the visit and the duration of each meal for each dog.

The aim of this study was to describe the change in feeding patterns of the dogs during the course of toxicity studies and to assess the use of these feeding patterns as a potentially more sensitive parameter for the health status of the animals.

2.2 Definition of "wellbeing"

According to the **Swiss Animal Welfare Act** wellbeing means:

If the body is in physical and emotional harmony with itself and the environment in accordance with its innate living needs (movement, nutrition, care), the animal feels well. This fettle is also characterized as the absence of pain, suffering or injury. Regular signs of wellbeing are health and normal behavior in any circumstances (GOETSCHEL 1986)

A more precise definition of the animal's wellbeing could be found in **The Guidelines of the Australian Government to promote the wellbeing of animals for scientific purposes 2008**. The guidelines can be referred to the experimental animals in Switzerland.

Animal wellbeing relates to evidence of how an animal is coping with a given situation and a judgment as to how the animal feels in these circumstances.
Wellbeing is an internal state of homeostasis and is influenced by internal and external factors. The factors can be distinguished between good and positive or bad and negative. Every animal has different demands, motivations, preferences and experiences wellbeing differently and individually. In addition, wellbeing in an animal can vary from time to time. Animals react with protective mechanisms to cope with a new situation and to adapt the internal state of homeostasis. If the animal is unable to cope with the internal or external factors, distress, disability, disease or death may result.

2.2.1 Physiological and behavioral indicators of wellbeing

Animals try to adapt themselves to the environmental conditions using behavioral and physiological mechanisms. These mechanisms are limited and individual for each animal.
To be able to assess the animals' condition, knowledge of species-specific behavior is important. Animal keepers have to be familiar with individual reactions to different situations of the animals to interpret their wellbeing.
Species-specific cage size and structure, light, sounds, ventilation etc. are important for a comfortable environment and the wellbeing of the animals. Conditions that are good for one species do not have to be good for another species.
Changes of the behavioral manner are often the first reaction to a new situation and can also show how well an animal is coping with stress factors.
The range and level of activities such as eating, drinking, playing, grooming, sleeping, resting, interactions with conspecifics and exploration of the environment can be used to describe patterns of behavior indicatives of the animal's wellbeing.
Species-specific differences will be seen in the types and levels of activities.
Indicators to asses an animal's state of health include general appearance, posture, coat condition, clinical signs (e.g. temperature, heart rate, respiratory rate), hematological and biochemical measurements, responses to handling, demeanor, temperament, maintenance of body weight (in immature animals, rate of weight gain) and reproductive performance (AUSTRALIAN GOVERNMENT 2008).

An animal is probably coping with its current situation, if the animal's physical needs, safety needs and psychological needs are provided (CLARK et al 1997) and no signs of disease or abnormal behavior are observed.

The following sensations: pain, suffer, injury, anxiety, and stress can influence the feeding behavior of dogs, most likely by decreasing the food intake and are therefore described more precisely in 2.2.2-2.2.6.

2.2.2 Pain

The International Association for the Study of Pain (IASP; www.iasp-pain.org) defines pain as "an unpleasant sensory and emotional experience associated with actual or potential tissue damage, or described in terms of such damage" (IASP 1979).
In animals, pain provokes a protective, motoric or vegetative reaction, which leads to avoiding such stimuli and also modifies their behavior (SANN 2000)
Nociceptors have a protective function and when being stimulated they trigger multiple physiological and behavioral responses. An unlearned response e.g. interruption of normal feeding or vocalization can be distinguished from learned responses e.g. turning its head from the noxious stimulus when, for example, heating the snout (CHAPMAN 1984).
Pain causes a trigger of these nociceptors in the body's tissue and signals are transferred to the central nervous system. The brain processes the signals and generates responses, interacting with the peripheral nervous system.
Nociceptors are localized in the skin, but also in muscles, joints, and viscera and in almost all organs in the body except for the central nervous system (SANN 2000).

Due to the lack of any direct means of communication in animals, a large amount of experiments were performed to measure pain e.g. heat, mechanical, electrical and chemical stimulation procedures (CHAPMAN 1984).
Variation in pain scores between observers, but also the subjective sensations of pain deliver unreliable results (FLECKNELL 1994). Clinical parameters like heart rate, respiration, and blood pressure were observed to increase during pain stimulus.
The aversiveness to pain depends on its duration and intensity. Animals accept acute pain lasting only for a short time better than chronic pain. Chronic pain can lead to pathological changes and influence the animal's wellbeing (NATIONAL RESEARCH COUNCIL 2008)
People conclude from their perception of pain to the animal and may misinterpret the animal's expressions of pain, e.g. screaming, howling, yelping, compressing the jaw, grinding of teeth, sweating, unmotivated turning or bending, licking of painful spots, trembling.
Pigs for example already scream when trying to catch them, while horses almost never scream. Some animals such as fish are not able to show pain, what does not mean they do not feel it (SAMBRAUS, STEIGER 1997)
What causes pain in humans does not have to do so in animals and conversely. It cannot be assumed that what does not cause pain in humans is also not felt as pain for animals.

2.2.3 Suffering

Suffering is the experience of negative emotions that is contrary to the animal's nature, the self preservation- and species preservation instincts.
Restriction of physical or by withdrawal of natural species friendly environment such as missing of nutrition and water can cause suffering. Social reasons such as isolation or overcrowding, illness can induce suffering as well as pain (GOETSCHEL 1986). The difference between pain and suffering can be explained by including all terms of aversion feelings which cannot be referred to the term of exact pain (SAMBRAUS, STEIGER 1997). Suffering can cause behavioral change or maladjustment, for example stereotypical behavior or lethargy.

2.2.4 Injury
Injury causes physical or psychological damage and can occur as a cause, an accompanying effect or a consequence of pain and suffering. It can be of physical or emotional nature e.g. if kept in a restricted space, which can be observed in animals kept in zoos (GOETSCHEL 1986).
Examples for injuries are lethargy, emaciation, dullness of sense organs, infertility, behavioral damage, weight loss or vertigo. (SAMBRAUS, STEIGER 1997)

2.2.5 Anxiety
Anxiety is an unpleasant emotional state when expecting a strong negative experience. The symptoms of sensation especially in mammals are basically the same as in humans. Examples are mydriasis, increased heart rate and breathing, hair bristle, sweating attacks, muscle tremor, chatter, increased or sudden urination and defecation (GOETSCHEL 1986).

2.2.6 Stress
Stress is the response of the animal to a 'stressor', which can be induced by external or internal factors, including pain. Stress is a normal feature of life, serving important adaptive functions (AUSTRALIAN GOVERNEMT 2008).
Stressors can be caused by viral or bacterial infection, threat of physical harm, hunger, and thirst.
Stressors are not necessarily adverse, they can also be pleasurable, e.g. exercise.

Stress is a real or perceived perturbation to an organism's physiological homeostasis or psychological wellbeing. In its *stress response,* the body uses behavioral, autonomic, neuroendocrine (release of glucocorticoids, prolactin) and immunological reactions. The factors do not have to be from an aversive stimulus to cause stress. Whenever a demand is asked from an animal it reacts and activates its inner resources (O'HEARE 2009).

Normal well managed stress situations are also defined as eustress or positive stimulus. Negative stress is also called distress and occurs when the body cannot cope with the assault of one or more stressors, depending on stressor duration, stressor intensity and the capacity of the individual animal to respond (AUSTRALIAN GOVERNMENT 2008). The animal is no longer able to bring its organism into physiological and/or psychological homeostasis (NATIONAL RESEARCH COUNCIL 2008).

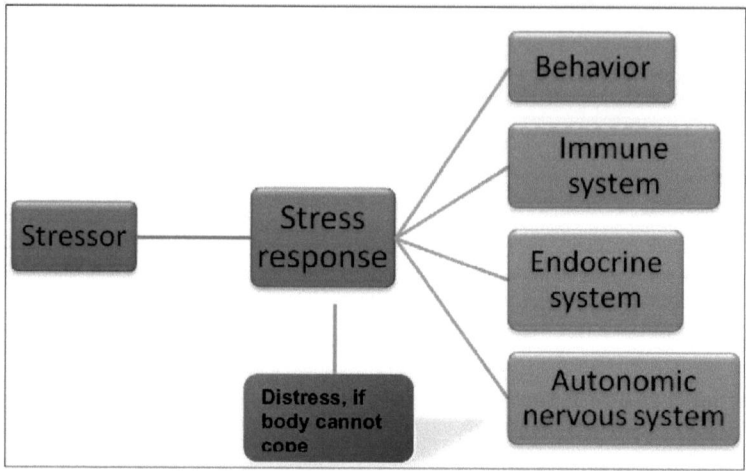

Figure 2.1: Model of stress and distress

Distress does not always appear as clear maladaptive behavior, such as abnormal feeding or aggression, but instead subclinical pathological changes, such as hypertension and immunosuppression can be measured (NATIONAL RESEARCH COUNCIL 2008).

2.3 Physiological measure of stress and distress

Behavior: Clinical signs of stress or distress:
- Increased heart rate and/or respiration rate
- Vomiting and/or diarrhea
- Slow motion movements
- Appeasement gestures
- Freeze
- Sitting down or lying down
- Changes in body weight
- Changes in food consumption

Endocrine system: Hypothalamic-pituitary-adrenal axis reacts to stress by releasing glucocorticoids, which are indicators for the impact and strength of a stressor. Glucocorticoid-release causes energy mobilization and is regulated by a negative feedback-loop, when stressor is removed or the animal has adapted to it.
Other stress hormones such as prolactin, growth hormone or luteinizing hormone (LH) can be used as well to monitor stress reactions (NATIONAL RESEARCH COUNCIL 2008)
Animals are capable to adapt to acute stress. Chronic stress causes an ongoing high level of circulating glucocorticosteroids, which can suppress secretion of growth hormone to inhibit growth, metabolic exhaustion from breakdown of skeletal muscle, suppression of T-lymphocyte activity ending in a higher risk of infections and finally death (WINGFIELD et al 1999).
Autonomic nervous system: The sympathetic system is activated by stressors and manifests in increased heart rate, redistribution of blood vessels to skeletal muscles (JÄNIG 1990).

Immunological parameters: The immune system is either activated, especially when acute stress occurs or it can also be suppressed, monitored with chronic stress (NATIONAL RESEARCH COUNCIL 2008). For example leukocytes are very high in the hematology results when taking blood from a cat or dog that is in an acute situation, but are usually decreased when checking blood of animals suffering from a chronic disease. (AUSTRALIAN GOVERNMENT 2008)

Even though most studies of stress reactions in animals are performed with mice, these pathways of stress reactions were also shown in dogs (BEERDA et al 1997, GALOSY 1979).

2.4 Severity grade of the constraint of the dog

Caused stress to animals due to interventions or measures during animal testing are divided into four categories, defined by the **Swiss Animal Welfare Act**:

2.4.1 No distress: Severity Grade 0

Interventions and manipulations in animals for experimental purposes as a result of which the animals experience no distress
(No pain, suffering, or injury)
Examples: withdrawal of blood samples for diagnostic purposes in cows; the housing of rats in enriched environments for behavioral observations

2.4.2 Minor distress: Severity Grade 1

Interventions and manipulations in animals for experimental purposes which subject the animals to a brief episode of minor distress (pain or injury)
Examples: injection of a drug requiring the use of restraint; castration of male animals under anesthesia

2.4.3 Moderate distress: Severity Grade 2

Interventions and manipulations in animals for experimental purposes which subject the animals to a brief episode of moderate distress, or a moderately long to long-lasting episode of minor stress (pain, suffering, or injury, extreme anxiety, or significant impairment of the general condition)
Examples: surgical treatment of a bone fracture on one leg that was purposely induced under anesthesia; castration of female animals (under anesthesia)

2.4.4 Severe distress: Severity Grade 3

Interventions and manipulations in animals for experimental purposes which cause the animals severe to very severe distress, or subject them to a moderately long to long-lasting episode of moderate distress
Examples: transplantations, potentially lethal infectious diseases

3. General behavior of dogs

Dogs are members of the order Carnivora and were the first species of animals to be domesticated about 15,000 years ago.
Dogs are social animals with a complex social ranking. Males are more aggressive towards other male dogs than females (VAN ZUTPHEN et al. 1993)
To interpret a dog's health status, not only the clinical signs should be monitored, but also their body language has to be familiar when working with them.

3.1. Behavioral signals

The general impression of a dog is described by body posture, mimic, sounds and expression (ROHN 2007).
Examples for body signals
- Relaxed:
    o relaxed muscles and posture
    o lively friendly view
    o calm and evenly ear movements
- scared:
    o taut or hunched pose
    o tail between legs
    o panting
    o hypersalivation
    o barking

3.2 Feeding behavior of dogs: General facts

The physiology of the feeding behavior of dogs is not as well documented as in rats and mice and therefore general statements about dogs have to be made carefully in this respect (HART 1995).
Similar to other species, there is a physiological correlation between meal size and the intermeal intervals, and obviously between metabolic body mass and energy intake.
In dogs, the daily caloric requirement can be digested and absorbed within 12 hours.
Dogs with free access to food eat several times a day, resulting in eating ⅔ to ¾ of the total energy intake during the active part of the day/night cycle (LANGHANS et al 2000).
RASHOFFE et al (1984) showed that Beagle dogs living outdoors under normal weather conditions and with free access to food ate on average three times a day, in the morning, afternoon and at dusk, but also whenever fresh food was offered. As expected, they ate more during cold season and less during the summer months.

Eating is controlled by a variety of physiological factors, but several non physiological factors also play a role in the daily energy intake of dogs.
High temperatures, estrus, illness (e.g. fever) or pain are examples that lower food intake whereas low temperature, high activity, rivalry, metabolic disorders, e.g. hyperthyroidism, malassimilation syndromes, or pregnancy cause higher daily intake (KITCHELL 1989)

Due to the large range of breed-specific body size and constitution, the variation of the maintenance energy requirement is much bigger in dogs than in other domestic animals. Different breeds vary not only in body size and weight, but also in spontaneous activity and type (KIENZLE E. et al 1991). To give just an example, in short haired dogs, the upper limit of thermic neutrality temperature is around 25 degrees; compared to fourteen degrees in long haired dogs (MUSSA et al 2005).
In general, many dogs are capable of controlling their energy intake and keep their body weight in good balance. However some dogs, e.g. Beagles, Retrievers and others tend to become obese if fed ad libitum, in particular when fed a palatable diet. (BRADSHAW 1991)

3.2.1 Palatability of the food: taste texture, and smell

Dogs use both taste and smell for their food selection (BRADSHAW 1991)
The taste system of dogs has some distinct aspects that differ from those found in rats and other omnivores or in herbivores. In general dogs' sensitivity to sodium is greater than in other mammalian groups like herbivores, but breed specific differences may exist. Beagle dogs e.g. seem to have only little preference for salt. (FREGLY 1980)

Dogs prefer wet or semidried diet to dry food, canned to freshly cooked food, cooked meat to raw meat, and novel flavor to familiar food. Like most mammals, dogs seem to have an innate preference for sucrose in liquids or solid food, and they seem to prefer fructose and lactose over sucrose (KITCHELL 1972).

Olfaction plays also an important role in food selection. Dogs can e.g. discriminate one meat from another by odor and dogs seem to prefer beef over horse meat. Consequently anosmic dogs do not have preferences for one meat over the other, but they can still distinguish between a diet containing sugar to a non-meat bland diet (HOUPT 1981)

3.3 Control of the digestion and food intake

The gastrointestinal tract is controlled by two nervous systems, the autonomic nervous system with the sympathetic and the parasympathetic part, and the enteric nervous system (EWE et al 1990).

Visceral afferent stimuli transmit information from the gut to the brain and the autonomic nervous system (sympathetic and parasympathetic) delivers signals from the brain to the gut. Parasympathetic activation has a prosecretoric effect by activating enteric pathways with a prosecretoric function. The vagus nerve innervates excitatory and inhibitory enteric motoneurons. The excitatory nerve cells release neurotransmitters which activate motoneurons over muscarinic effectors. In contrary, the inhibitory effect is based on the release of neurotransmitters that have an inhibiting effect on the effector cells. The sympathetic stimuli have an inhibiting effect on secretion and peristalsis (SCHEMANN 2000)

The enteric nervous system is the main part of the control of the digestive process and is separated into two parts, i.e. into the myenteric plexus, which mainly innervates the muscular part, and the submucosal plexus which mainly controls absorption und secretion.
Three different types of neurons exist within the enteric nervous system; these are sensoric neurons, interneurons and motoneurons.
Sensoric neurons register either wall tension (mechanoreceptors) or react to chemical stimuli (chemoreceptors).
Interneurons are responsible for the communication between the enteric neurons, hence, signals from sensoric or interneurons are transferred to the motoneurons and their activation can cause an excitation or an inhibition at the effector cells (e.g. smooth muscle cell or secretory cell) (SCHEMANN 2000).

Neurotransmitters like acetylcholine or substance P have a stimulating effect on the (muscular) motoneurons while nitric oxide (NO), vasoactive intestinal polypeptide (VIP) and adenosine triphosphate (ATP) cause a relaxation of the intestine. Secreto-motoneurons are activated by acetylcholine and VIP and inhibited by somatostatin and neuropeptid Y (NPY). These mechanisms are very important for coordination of the peristaltic process. Uptake of food activates a regulatory circuit. Wall tension activates sensoric neurons, which in turn activate motoneurons. Aboral of the stimulus, the motoneurons cause a relaxation, oral to the stimulus, they cause a contraction. The physiological program that controls peristalsis is modulated by pathologic peristaltic processes, e.g. due to metabolic or infectious diseases or intoxication. They can result in hypoperistalsis and atonic intestines or in diarrhea as a symptom of hyperperistalsis (SCHEMANN 2000).

The enteric neurons are in close contact with the enteric immune system. Immune cells release histamine, prostaglandins or leucotrienes which activate motor and mucosal reflexes; these typically result in increased secretion and motor function with the aim to dilute toxins and to strain the digestive tract faster (SCHEMANN 2000).
These interactions are a potentially important aspect relevant for toxicity studies, because some substances can cause lymphoid depletion and therefore influence this neuro-immune-interaction.

3.3.1 Central mechanism

The hypothalamus is a very important neural center for the control of food intake (KITCHELL 1989).
Together with the brain stem, the hypothalamus controls the fundamental aspects of eating. Both parts also interconnect with the limbic system which contributes to hedonic aspects in eating control. Details about the brain centers involved in the control of eating go far beyond the scope of this work and only few aspects will be mentioned briefly.

Afferent vagal fibers transmit the signals from the gastrointestinal and hepatic sensors to the solitary tract nucleus (NTS) of the medulla oblongata which interacts with the hypothalamus, the limbic system and also the cerebral cortex (LANGHANS et al 2000).
The area postrema (AP) has a partially open blood brain barrier and acts as a chemoreceptor area for substances circulating in the blood. The AP is in close communication with the NTS; together, constitute the primary central input area for a large number of peripheral signals involved in the control of eating (LANGHANS et al 2000).

3.3.2 Hunger, satiety and satiation

SCHMIDT et al (1979) defined hunger as the need to consume food. It is a general sensation where different mechanisms are involved; the physiological mechanisms inducing hunger are still largely unknown.

Glucose may play an important role in eliciting hunger. Glucose is the most important energy source for cells, and in particular for the brain. The glucostatic theory claims that decreased availability of glucoses causes the feeling of hunger (SCHMIDT 1979).

GEOGHEGAN et al (1995) described satiety as a psychophysical phenomenon produced by signals arising from different stages of the digestive and absorptive process. If too much food has been eaten, the feeling of fullness appears. In the more current view and in terms of physiological controls, one differentiates between "satiation" signals that control meal size by determining meal ending satiation, and "satiety" signals that control the onset of a subsequent meal. The former signals are much better identified than the latter.
Preabsorptive (stomach distension) and postabsorptive signals (hormones e.g. cholecystokinin) during the digestive process that influence the meal size can be distinguished (SCHMIDT1979), which are explained in 3.3.3 – 3.3.4.
Another factor that needs to be taken into account is a drop of palatability of the diet during the meal. This effect is only specific for that particular diet eaten. If another taste of food is offered, the animal (or human) will reinitiate or continue to eat.
This gustatory specific effect could be important in feral living animals to obtain a well balanced nutrition when switching from one nutritive source to another (LANGHANS et al 2000)

3.3.3 Gastrointestinal control

In an experiment by JANOWITZ and GROSSMAN M.I (1949), dogs were fitted with a gastric fistula to remove or add food to the stomach before or during mealtime. Meal size was smaller, if food was added and was bigger, if food was removed
Further studies showed that stomach distension during a meal sends afferent signals to the NTS and from there to the brain and limits meal size, proportional to the degree of gastric

wall stretch (CHENG et al 1993). This mechanism is independent from the diets' nutritive value; inert material is just as effective as a high caloric diet. Hence, meal size may in part be determined by gastric distension, but the exact physiological relevance of this effect is still under debate.

3.3.3.4 Gastric small bowel signals:
The presence and absorption of nutrients from the small intestine influences the propagation of food from the stomach to the small intestine via vagal and hormonal processes by a feedback regulatory circuit.
Many gut hormones influence food intake directly or indirectly; the majority of the hormones have an inhibiting effect on food intake (CHAUDHRI et al 2006).
One of the major hormones controlling food intake and gastric emptying is cholecystokinin (CCK). The NTS is the primary relay station within the brain that processes satiation induced by CCK. CCK, together with a number of other gastrointestinal hormones (e.g., amylin, glucagon, ghrelin, Intestinal glucagon-like peptide) seems to be the major player in meal size control (LUTZ 2006). This is also corroborated by a number of studies in dogs
CCK reduces eating, but not total food intake (LUTZ 2006). High doses of CCK lead to vomiting in dogs (LEVINE et al. 1984).SIMMONS et al (1998) describe the longer lasting effect of inhibiting food by a CCK peptide analog (ARL 15849) in dogs compared to CCK-8 peptide which may be useful in the treatment of eating disorders.

3.3.4 Metabolic and neurochemical Influence on satiety
Intestinal sensors for glucose, amino acids and fatty acids as well as neurotransmitters triggered by these nutrients are also involved in the process of food intake control.
Glucose sensors in the periphery (e.g. hepatic portal vein), but also in the central nervous system, especially in the medulla oblongata seem to be involved. It is not fully understood how glucose exactly influences eating, however it is well established that glucose antimetabolites have a stimulating influence on food intake, whereas a glucose infusion, at least under certain conditions decreases food intake (LANGHANS, SCHARRER 2000).
The sensors for oxidized fatty acids are especially located in the liver and perhaps in the small intestinal mucosa and play an important role in maintenance of satiety (LANGHANS, SCHARRER 2000).
The main role of metabolic signals may be that their prolonged activation compared to gastrointestinal signals contributes to the maintenance of the satiety after a meal

3.3.5 Polyphagia and Anorexia
Changes in the feeding behavior of dogs such as anorexia or hyperphagia are well known symptoms in clinical practice, which are noticed early on by the pets' owners.
Anorexia can be complete or partial, and it can be expressed as showing no interest in food and be due to environmental stress, such as moving, new animals, regrouping or new people. However, it can also be due to illness and a decreased wellbeing due to local effects of the gastrointestinal system, metabolic derangements, pain, and central neural lesions or generally in many severe disease states.
Interestingly, anorexia or reduced food intake during the acute phase of a disease are also part of the host's defense mechanism and may in fact be beneficial for survival early in the disease process (HART 1988).
Cytokines such as interleukin-1, tumor necrosis factor-alpha (TNF-α) and interferon-γ inhibit food intake and most likely play important roles in such situations (LANGHANS 2004). LANGHANS et al (2007) could show that administration of the bacterial endotoxin lipopolysaccharides (LPS), which is often used to model infectious disease states, inhibits eating by reducing the number of daily meals. LPS stimulates the production of cytokines that then act on the brain to inhibit feeding.

On the other extreme, polyphagia is defined as excessive consumption of food and is a more specific symptom, it can be physiologic e.g. due to increased energy turnover, or pathologic e.g. metabolic disorders, such as hyperthyroidism or exocrine pancreas insufficiency (EPI) (KITCHELL 1989).

3.3.6 Taste Aversion

Taste preference or aversion is the acceptance or refusal of food intake influenced by innate and acquired responses, also called the unconditioned stimulus (US)
Innate reflexes are based on fixed neuronal connections between receptors and effectors. An innate taste aversion for bitter and an innate taste preference for sweet food exist in most species. Interestingly, innate taste preferences can change, e.g. the palatability for a taste during the meal decreases and increases for another taste (LANGHANS et al 2000).

For acquired reflexes, the connection between receptors and effectors is formed by learning processes. Theses reflexes are also called "conditioned" reflexes (CS) (SCHMIDT 1990). When a novel taste is followed by general reduction of the animal's wellbeing or a visceral illness (unconditional stimulus), the animal associates the illness with the food and avoids this taste. This is also called **conditioned taste aversion (CTA)**. CTA can be induced, even though the decrease in wellbeing may be completely unrelated with the meal. In fact many hours may intervene between the CS and the US, and a CTA can still be formed. CTA can also develop if the animal is asleep, anesthetized or in coma when the US is administered (REILLY 2005)
To give just an example, administration of LPS as an unconditioned stimulus leads to a learned taste aversion; taste aversion can lead to anorexia when no other food is available (WEINGARTEN et al 1993)
Taste aversion may be difficult to differentiate from anorexia caused by other reasons, e.g. metabolic diseases, if only one diet is available.

3.4 Drug discovery and development process – an Overview

The human patient is the main focus and the drug discovery and development process is designed to ensure that innovative new medicine are effective, safe and available for patients in the shortest possible time to help them overcome a disease and improve their lives.
Before a new drug is available on the market, several steps have to be fulfilled to guarantee the drugs' safety and efficacy (NOVARTIS PHARMA).

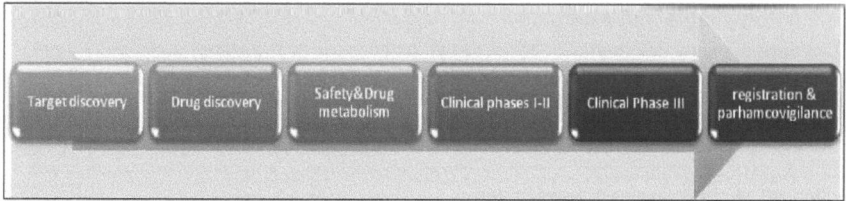

Figure 3.4: Process of drug development

3.4.1 Target discovery

In a first step to treat a disease, its mechanism has to be discovered and understood. It is important to know, which genes are involved and how they are altered, how they affect the proteins they encode and what effect it has on living cells and organs of the patient's body. Once the scientists have found the proteins that play a main role in the disease outbreak, they have to select a target for the new medicine. A target is generally a single molecule, such as a gene or protein, which is involved in a particular disease (DRUG DISCOVERY, http://www.innovation.org/drug_discovery/objects/pdf/RD_Brochure.pdf)

3.4.2 Drug discovery
Computer animated design and high-throughput screening are used to find chemical compounds of biologics (mostly molecules) that bind to and act on the identified target which causes an alteration of the protein and therefore of the disease.
From the discovery to the registration of a new drug, it takes around fourteen years with costs of two billion dollars. Only one out of 10,000 tested compounds reaches the market.

3.4.3 Safety and drug metabolism
If a potential new drug (compound) is found, series of tests have to be performed to provide an early assessment to the safety of the compound. It is important to know the compounds pharmacological behavior that means how it is absorbed, distributed, metabolized, and excreted. Based on this knowledge, toxicological effects can be discovered and toxicological doses are defined in dose selection studies.
While pharmacological tests are performed to understand the compounds behavior inside the body, toxicological tests are necessary for its safety and to target organ toxicity (DRUG DISCOVERY, http://www.innovation.org/drug_discovery/objects/pdf/RD_Brochure.pdf).

Even though, most tests can be performed on computer based simulations, complex diseases can mostly only be understood to the use of animal studies. One step closer to drug safety is detecting any toxic effects on target organs in animals and directing the attention to organ-related biomarkers to survey the process.
Furthermore, the Government or the health authorities require that drugs are tested in animals before tested in humans to help assure their safe use.
It is not completely answered, how well animal studies predict the response overall of humans. Not all adverse effects observed in animals occur in humans and vice versa, but there is a higher concordance of toxicity of pharmaceuticals in humans and animals when tested in rodents and non-rodents than only tested in one species (OLSON et al 2000).
The concordance is especially seen in hematological, gastrointestinal, and cardiovascular toxicity effects.

As already mentioned, pharmaceuticals must be tested in animals, normally in rodent and non-rodent species.
The selection to choose the most appropriate animal in animal tests is based on regulatory requirements, ethics, the scientific requirement to obtain the best possible prediction of the human response and animal husbandry.
The Association of the British Pharmaceutical Industry (ABPI) in conjunction with the UK Home Office published a paper in 2002 with "points to consider" when selecting species for animal tests.
Some important points are listed here:

- Species selection should be based on similarity to humans of an aspect of anatomy and/or physiology which is likely to be relevant to the pharmacological or toxic response to the compound. Important to know pharmacokinetic profile, including biotransformation and conversion of pro-drug to active substances
- Wherever possible selected species should respond to the primary pharmacodynamic effect of the substance
- Similarity to human toxicity for that substance based on in vitro data and/or related compounds already given to humans
- Availability of background data which is especially important to help distinguish treatment-related pathological effects from spontaneous findings
- For the safety assessment program early in vitro and in vivo studies are used to help select the species. In most cases, the dog is effectively the default species, driven by historical data/experience, practicalities, legislative requirements and availability

The dog has been used for animal tests for a long time resulting in extensive knowledge and understanding around the use of dogs.

3.4.4 Clinical trial I-II
In clinical trial I 20-100 healthy volunteers are tested to determine the drug's safety and pharmacological kinetics and dynamics.
In clinical trial II, the drug is tested in 100-250 patients with the disease to evaluate its efficacy as well as its safety and side effects and determine optimal doses (NOVARTIS PHARMA).

3.4.5 Clinical trial III
1000-3000 or more patients are tested for the investigation of the new drug and to monitor side effects. Significant data about safety, efficacy and the overall benefit-risk-relationship of the new drug are statistically generated (NOVARTIS PHARMA).

3.4.6 Registration and Pharmacovigilance
When all three phases are successfully achieved, the new drug application can be handed in to the health authority (Swissmedic in Switzerland, Food&Drug Administration in USA). The health authority reviews all the information and can approve the application, if the medicine is considered safe and effective.

3.5 Different kind of studies in toxicology

3.5.1 Compound selection studies
Compound selection studies are used to evaluate toxicological effect of the potential drug in unison with pharmacological investigations, mostly at the end of the compound selection phase

3.5.2 Dose selection studies
Dose selection studies are performed to deliver appropriate information on the characteristics of the test compound in non-rodents and identify the appropriate dose levels for the regulatory toxicity studies, thus achieving the most effective use of the animals (SMITH et al 2004)

3.5.2.1 Rising dose study
Rising dose studies are necessary to detect a tolerance limit based on the results of an in vivo test, following the administration of single, escalating doses of test chemical (SMITH et al 2004)

3.5.2.2 Dose range finding study
Dose range finding studies are performed to identify a tolerance limit following the repeated administration of the highest feasible dose based on the outcome of a rising dose study for subsequent regulatory studies.

3.5.3 Regulatory studies
- Regulatory studies are required for clinical trial I in men and are performed under good laboratory practice (GLP) regulations
- The main objective is to establish potential hazards associated with the test item by identifying organ toxicity.
- GLP is a quality safety system to survey the organization, process, documentation, archiving and reporting of relevant non-clinical medical- and environmental safety studies for pharmaceutical drugs tested in testing animals or in vitro

3.6 Aim of this study

In my research study, I want to determine the normal feeding behavior of untreated laboratory dogs during the pretest and to create a feeding profile for comparison with the application phase to observe deviations from the normal feeding pattern and to identify the effects of the test item at an early stage. In this way, I hope to identify a drug-induced effect on the dogs' state of health at an early stage.

4. Materials und Methods

4.1 Animals

Novartis uses purebred intact female and male Marshall Beagles, bred in Italy and shipped to Novartis when they are about eight to ten months old.
The dogs were vaccinated against canine distemper, infectious canine hepatitis, parainfluenza, leptospirosis, parvovirus, adenovirus, coronavirus, and rabies and went through antiparasitic therapy at the supplier.
At the beginning of the studies, dogs had an average age between ten to thirteen months and the average weight for females was 8.9kg and for males was 10.8kg.

4.1.1 Procedure from the first entry of dogs to the end of the study

After arriving at Novartis animal husbandry, the animals have to pass a health check to examine the general health condition of the animals and to take the actual body weight. The dogs were chipped with the implant on the right side of the neck to access the feeder (see below). Feces samples for microbiological analysis were sent to the laboratory.

For the first few weeks, they stay in the quarantine section to acclimatize to the new environment and the new feeding system; recommended are at least seven days to acclimatize (Working group of LASA, 2005). All dogs are fed with the same amount of 450g and same brand (Provimi-Kliba, Kaiseraugst) of complete dry dog food. Certain dogs lost weight even with the amount of 450g, thus they received a higher daily food limit.

If no symptoms or problems are observed and the entry examination is normal, dogs are moved to a new floor, where they have another few weeks to acclimatize before they are divided into the study groups. The guidelines for the transport of laboratory animals recommend at least another three days of adaption time, when moving the animals to a new building In the new rooms, the dogs have unlimited access to an outdoor balcony area.

The study itself starts with a pretest period with different in-life examinations to evaluate the baselines of the dogs and to test their applicability for the study. Inappropriate animals e.g. due to uncooperative behavior or medical issues are exchanged.
Three to five dogs of the same dosing group and gender are group housed, depending on how many animals are needed for the individual studies.

Animals will be separated to facilitate recording of clinical signs, conduct of special investigations and/or to avoid aggressive behavior.

During the study, various tests or samples are taken (explained under 4.3).
At the end of the study, the dogs are normally euthanized for macroscopic and microscopic pathology examinations.

4.2 Housing facilities

Animals are group housed in pens ($2m^2$/animal) which can be separated with a movable grid, if necessary.

Each of these pens has a water nipple for *ad libitum* tap water access and an elevated platform with a privacy shield toward the other pen, toys, and granulated bedding material. Radio is playing at low volume from 6am to 6pm.

The feeding machines are installed between the third and the fourth pen (see figure 4.1 and 4.2) with two accesses on opposite sides where dogs can eat from 10am to 11pm.

The dogs have free access to the balcony through a flap door. In this way the animals are exposed to weather conditions and the normal 24-hours light-dark cycle. In addition to natural daylight cycle, fluorescent light for a 12-hour light/12-hour dark cycle is guaranteed.

Rees Environmental Monitoring System (EnRep) is installed in the rooms to control the temperature, light and humidity. The target range is set to 18-22°C and 40-70% humidity. Longer deviations from the target ranges will be noticed and set off an alarm.

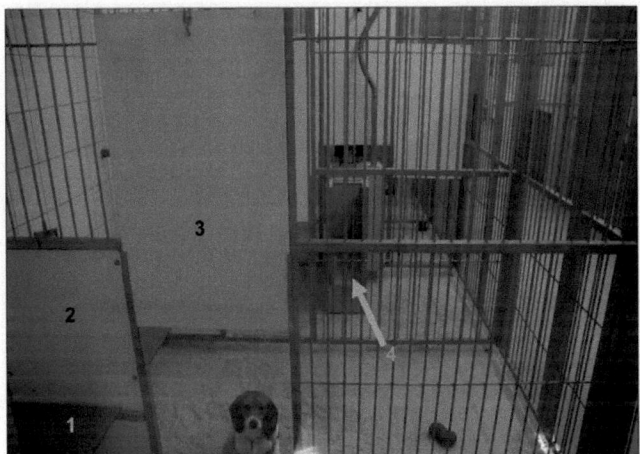

Figure 4.1: Dog room from the front : *1= elevated platform, 2= privacy shield, 3= movable grid, 4= entrance to feeder*

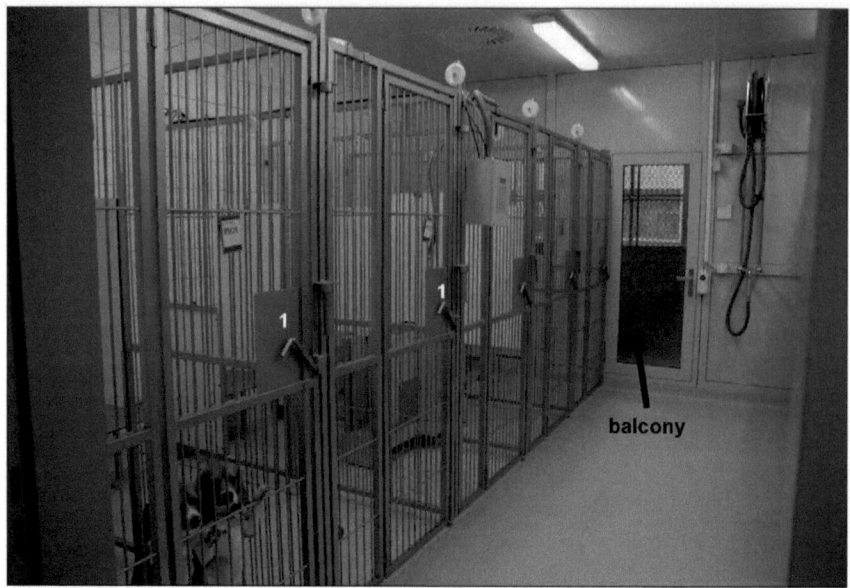

Figure 4.2: Dog room from the side: *1= door opener*

In figure 4.2, the single pens are distinguishable by the door openers. The black arrow points to the balcony.

4.3 Study data material

In 2007, Novartis moved from one building to a new location with new husbandry conditions. To have the same conditions throughout my analysis, only studies after the relocation were considered. In addition, certain criterions had to be fulfilled:
- At least three animals per group
- Duration of the study had to be longer than one week
- All three phases (pretest, main phase and recovery phase) should be evaluated
- Measurable deviations of the food consumption during the study performance should be noted in the majority of the studies
- Symptoms had to have been noted in some of the studies

Considering these criteria, sixteen studies between 2007 and 2010 were chosen, which included 459 dogs; 227 females and 232 males.

Three of these sixteen studies did not have a recovery phase, but with no consequences for the evaluation of the feeding behavior.

One study of the sixteen studies had only a main phase of two weeks instead of four weeks.

In one study, five dose groups existed, but group 5 was not included into the evaluation.

The chosen studies are all regulatory studies that ran under the same circumstances and the same living conditions.

4.4 Structure of a regulatory-study

Only regulatory -studies were used for this analysis and therefore only the structure of this type of study will be explained in more detail. In general (exceptions see above), the studies have a one week pretest phase, followed by a four week main phase and a four week recovery phase. One of the objectives of the one month studies is to allow dose selection for longer term regulatory studies (LASA 2009).
The study is separated into three phases:

- Pretest
- Main phase = treatment phase
- Recovery phase

4.4.1 Pretest

The duration of the pretest is normally seven days. The dogs are randomly separated into their dose groups at the beginning of the pretest and allocated to new rooms.
During this week, baseline data of all dogs are evaluated by collecting blood and urine samples, performing electrocardiograms (ECG) and ophthalmoscopic examinations as well as other tests listed in 4.5. Baseline data is important for the comparison with the findings during the studies or to identify and exchange an inappropriate animal due to inappropriate baseline results.
During the pretest, dogs can acclimatize to the new rooms and the new group members.

The dogs are separated into four groups:

- Control group 1: dosed with a placebo, normally five animals of both sexes
- Low dose group 2: normally three animals of both sexes are dosed with test substance in a dose where no side effects are expected
- Middle dose group 3: normally three animals of both sexes are dosed with an intermediate dosage of the test substance
- High dose group 4: normally five animals of both sexes are dosed with the highest possible dose that is tolerated for the study duration. The maximum tolerated dose is determined on a previous study by parameters such as clinical signs and reductions in body weight and food consumption (LASA 2009)

Whenever possible, the number of animals used for studies is reduced to the minimum and groups may be reduced to two or three groups only instead of four groups. This depends on the information gained in prior tests.

4.4.2 Main phase = treatment phase

The duration of the main phase period is usually related to the duration, therapeutic indication and scale of the proposed clinical trial, commonly four weeks.

Table 4.1: Recommended duration of repeated-dose toxicity studies (EMeA 2009)

Duration of indicated treatment of clinical trial in humans	Rodents	Non-rodents
Up to two weeks	one month	one month
>two weeks to one month	three months	three months
>one month to three months	six months	six months
>three months	six months	nine months

The similar route of application is chosen to that intended for use in man.

Regularly, females and males of each dosing group share a room, males on one side and females on the other side. It is important that all animals are kept under the same conditions to exclude any environmental influence.

The main phase starts with the first application. Especially during the first three days, animals are distracted from their daily routine due to the start of daily examinations and applications. Blood samples for kinetics are taken several times in certain intervals within the first two days. Depending on the study, ECG and neurological examinations are executed.

Within the first three days of the main phase, it is not known what kind of symptoms appear and therefore, animals are kept separated after dosing for two to three hours to observe any potentially occurring symptoms. After the first three days of clinical observation and established symptoms, the animals do not need to be separated anymore and are grouped immediately after dosing.

During the whole main phase, symptoms are taken whenever possible and documented, but at least two times a day.

If not otherwise defined, body weight is taken twice weekly.

Normally, in-life examinations are taken again at the end of the phase during the last week. Depending on the study, the in-life examinations could be performed more than twice during the main phase.

At the end of the main phase, two animals of the control and high dose groups of both sexes continue to the recovery phase. The other animals are euthanized and send to pathology for necropsy.

4.4.3 Recovery

Usually two control and two high dose animals of each gender enter the recovery phase and are observed for another two to four weeks.

During this time, no examinations are made until the end of the phase, except for clinical observation. At the end of the four week phase, the animals go through the same examinations as at the beginning of the main phase (e.g. ECG, blood samples, and urine samples, but no TK blood sampling) and are then euthanized and send to pathology for necropsy.

4.5 In-life examinations

The various in-life examinations performed throughout the whole study are briefly described below:

4.5.1 Clinical observations

Clinical signs are assessed and scored if necessary e.g. neurological symptoms are described as slight to marked in appearance. Efforts are made to characterize onset and duration of signs observed. The observations are documented at least once a day

4.5.2 Body weight

Individual body weights are measured using an electronic balance. Normally body weight is measured twice a week. If weight loss is expected, body weight will be measured on a more frequent basis.

4.5.3 Food consumption

Daily values are recorded using an automated feeding system.

Dry food in pellet form is fed.

If a study causes anorexia or lower food intake, dry food is mixed with water and dogs are fed manually. Because most dogs prefer wet food to dry food, they start to eat the mixture.

Energy requirement for young laboratory animals:

The required metabolisable energy (ME) for dogs is multiplied with the metabolic body mass ($BM^{0.75}$) to calculate the energy requirement for the day (measured in calories). The required caloric value (Kcal) per kg $BM^{0.75}$ for young laboratory dogs is 140 Kcal or 0.59 mega joules (MJ) (GV-SOLAS).
The formula to calculate the required daily intake is:

Kcal ME* kg $BM^{0.75}$, 0.59 MJ ME * kg $BM^{0.75}$

For example, a 10 kg dog has a daily caloric need of 787kcal or 260g dry food per day. The Beagle dogs in Novartis used to receive 350g per day, but this amount seemed too low. Several animals lost body weight. Due to this observation, the daily food allowance was increased to 450g.

The major nutrients of the dogs' dry pellet food:

- Dry matter 88.0%
- Crude protein 22.5%
- Crude fat 6.0%
- Crude fiber 3.5%
- Crude ash 6.3%
- Nitrogen free extract (NFE) 49.7%
- Gross energy 16.7
- Starch 33%
- Ingredients: Flacked cereals, wheat, poultry meal, flacked oats, soybean meal, wheat middlings, soybean oil, wheat germ, corn, minerals, vitamins, amino acids

4.5.4 ECG

ECGs are recorded using the Cardiovit AT-60 cardiograph. The ECG traces are evaluated visually and the following parameters were measured: heart rate, PQ, QRS and QT intervals. Normally, ECG-recordings are taken during the pretest period to give predose background values, on day 2 of the main phase (usually at the Tmax) to monitor any cardiac effects soon after dosing, and 24hours after the second dose (day 3) to check for recovery from any effects seen on day 2.
Another two ECG-recordings are performed in the last weeks of the main phase to see any deviations after long term treatment (at Tmax and 24hours after dosing). At the end of the recovery phase another session of ECG-recordings are performed to compare the results with the ones of the main phase. In some cases, abnormal ECG-results occur during the main phase and may disappear in the recovery phase.

4.5.5 Ophthalmology

After instillation of a mydriatic, ophthalmological examinations are performed in a dark room, using a slit lamp and an indirect ophthalmoscope.
Any abnormalities are documented.

4.5.6 Neurology

Animals are carefully observed for gait anomalies with special consideration of activity, muscle coordination and wide stance of the hind legs, followed by functional testing.
The neurology test is only planned, if neurological symptoms are expected or if the test item is tested for neurological diseases such as Parkinson.

4.5.7 Clinical pathology: hematology, clinical biochemistry and urinalysis

Usually, animals have no access to food for at least 6 hours before blood or urine collection, but have free access to water. Blood specimens are taken from a peripheral vein before administration.

If required, blood samplings are also collected more frequently during the main phase, e.g. studies with immunosuppressive response.

4.5.7.1 Hematology
Blood specimens for analysis of the coagulation parameters are taken into sodium citrate anticoagulant; otherwise the blood is collected into ethylenediaminetetraacetic acid (EDTA) anticoagulant.
A total white and red blood cell profile is required during pretest, at the end of the main phase and at the end of the recovery.

4.5.7.2 Clinical biochemistry
Blood specimens for analysis are collected using no anticoagulant. Blood collection is required during the pretest, at the end of the main phase and at the end of the recovery to be able to compare any deviations.

4.5.7.3 Urinalysis
Urine is collected by catheterization. Normally urinalysis is done in the pretest, within the last week of the main phase and at the end of the recovery

4.5.9 Toxicokinetics and special investigation
While toxicokinetics is always required, special investigations such as gene and protein profiling can be required, depending on the use of the test item.
After the 1st and one of the last administrations, blood is taken from all main group animals at time points within 24 hours post-dose to calculate following parameters: maximum plasma concentration of the drug (C_{max}), C_{max}/dose, area under curve (AUC) (0-24h), AUC (0-24h)/dose, time after administration of a drug when C_{max} is reached (T_{max}).

4.5.10 Pathology
At the end of the study, the dogs are euthanized and a macroscopic organ evaluation is performed. Organs listed in the study plan are collected, specific organs are weighed and if other tissues show any macroscopic alterations, samples are taken for histology. A selected set of tissues are processed for histopathological examination.

4.6 Dog feeding system
The dog feeding system consists of three main parts

- Dog feeder: Feeding station with a silo on top
- Dogfeed: Display and control units of the dog feeder
- Software : to transfer recorded data from the control unit to the main server

4.6.1 Dog feeder
The feeding station is covered with plastic walls, which are framed with a steel rail at the ends for protection against being chewed up by the dogs. There are two entrances (figure 4.5 black arrows) on opposite sides and a sight protection to protect low-ranking dogs from dominant dogs, when former enters the feeder. A short passage leads the dogs to the feeding bowl.

The feeding bowl, placed on a precision balance, is accessible by 2 doors which open by electro-pneumatic valves. If a dog enters the feeding station, a transponder receiver registers its identification (ID) and sends the information about meal duration time, food intake, and number of visits to the server.

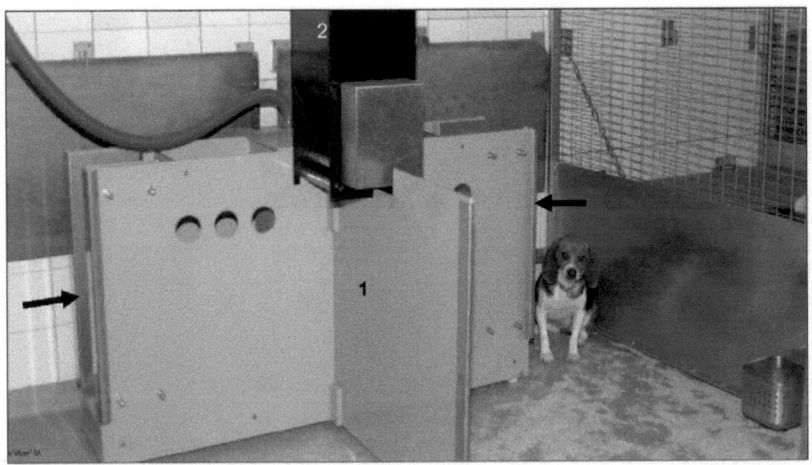

Figure 4.3: Dogfeeder from the outside: *Black arrows point to the entrances of the feeder, 1= side protection, 2: silo*

In figure 4.3, the entrances to the passages that lead to the food bowl are demonstrated. The dog on one side does not see when another dog enters the feeder on the opposite side due to the sight protection (1).

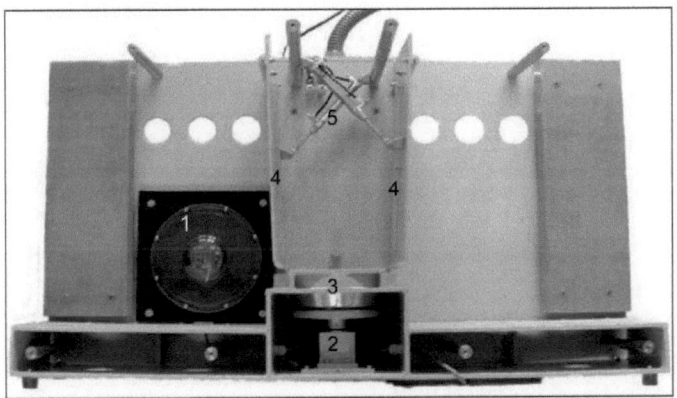

Figure 4.4: Inside part of the Dogfeeder: *1= transponder receiver, 2= Balance, 3= Food bowl, 4= Food access door, 5= electropneumatic pistons*

Picture 4.4 illustrates the hardware of the dog feeder from the inside. The food bowl (3) is placed in the middle over the balance (2) and the dogs can enter from left or right. The pneumatic pistons (5) open the food access doors (4) as soon as the transponder receiver (1) registers a dog in the passage.

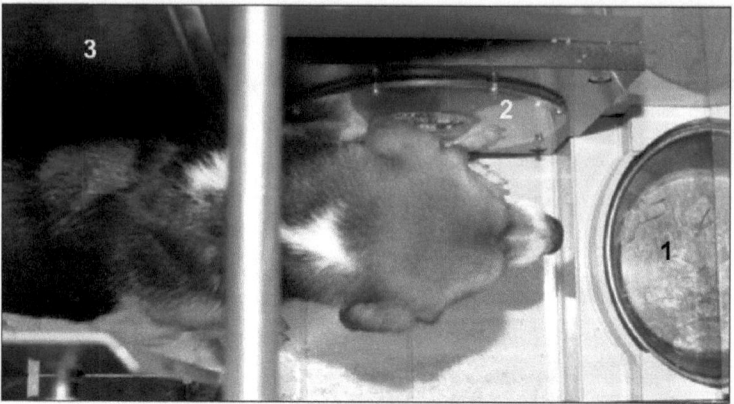

Figure 4.5: Food bowl and transponder receiver: *1= Food bowl, 2= transponder receiver, 3= Food access door*

From the top, it is shown how a dog gets to the food bowl. The receiver (2) on the left side in figure 4.5 is on the opposite side to that shown in figure 4.4. The transponder was originally implanted on the left side of the neck. Thereafter the dogs were required to have their identification chip implanted on the left side. This implant was not big enough to be read by the transponder receiver and the second chip for the dog feeder had to be implanted on the right side of the neck, resulting in changing the transponder receiver to the right side of the dog feeder.

4.6.2 Implant

The transponder for the animal ID is packed in glass and implanted subcutaneous on the right side of the neck.

The dogs must be registered at the feeding station to have access. Up to a maximum of ten animals for each dog feeder is possible, limited by the food silo, which would be emptied too fast by a larger group.

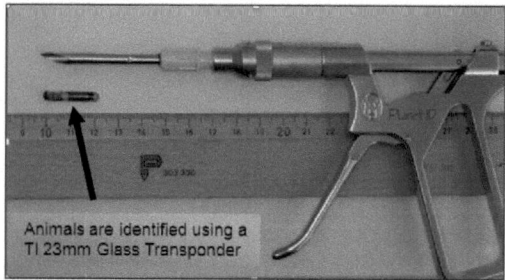

Figure 4.6: Implant: the black arrow points to the implant

4.6.3 Situations that may occur during the feeding process

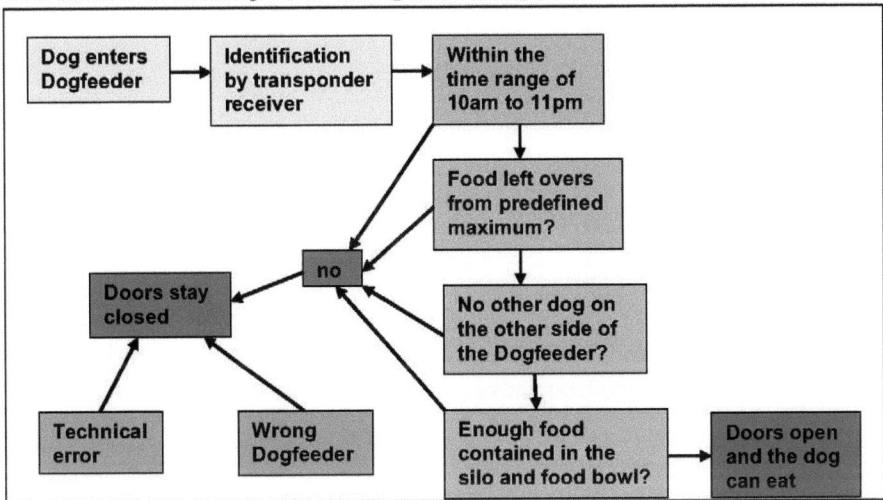

Figure 4.7: Required points to get access to the food bowl

Certain criteria have to be fulfilled before the dog can enter the dog feeder.
Figure 4.7 demonstrates the different steps the dog has to pass to get access to the food bowl.
First of all, the dog has to be registered at the feeder station. As a next step, the visit has to be within the time range. Then, the dog can only eat, if it has not yet eaten its entire allocated amount of food and if no other dog is eating at the same time on the other side.

The food intake of the dog can be interrupted by another dog which may enter the passage from the same side to push the former away. In this case, the doors close and the food that was eaten is accredited to the first dog.
Some dogs, particularly females, tend to sleep in the feeder passage, especially after they have eaten. This brings two disadvantages:
1. The recorded meal duration time is incorrect
2. Other dogs cannot eat from the opposite side

4.6.4 Display and control units

The control unit box, suspended on a hook, contains the control- and communication software dog feed.
On the visual display, the dog feeder can be switched to service mode to keep the doors closed or opened, e.g. for cleaning or to tare the balance.

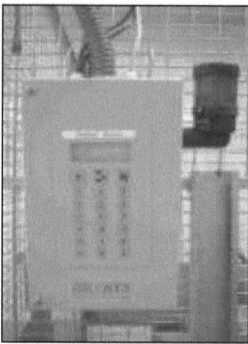

Figure 4.8: Display and control monitor

Other important functions of dog feed are:
- Network connectivity to the management software FeeditManager for communication
- Receive and perform instructions of feeding from FeeditManager
- Feeding of the registered animals in a 24-hour cycle
- Recording and saving all feeding data of each animal
- Register and set up alarm
- Transfer of all saved data to the database server

4.6.5 Meal Definition

Although meal patterns for animals like the rat or livestock have often been analyzed, there has been little uniformity in how meals have been defined for dogs.

Meals are normally conceptualized with two-process models (ZORRILLA et al 2005). A cluster of feeding events (intrameal intervals) presents the actual "meal" that is separated from other clusters by a non-feeding interval, the so called intermeal interval.

The various parameters that are evaluated in this research are:
- Daily food intake (DFI): the total amount of the single meals of one day
- Meal duration time (MDT): The occupation time they spent to eat the daily amount
- Number of visits per day (VpD): How many single meals per day
- Single meals of the day: average of the single meals during the day
- Single meal duration time: The time they spend for a single meal
- Timetable: On what time of day they eat

DEMARIA-PESCE et al (1996) mathematically investigated the various meal parameters in rats. The longest intrameal interval was fourteen mins (minutes), but most intrameal intervals lasted two mins. The intermeal intervals could last over 600 mins.

RASHOTTE et al (1984) determined the intermeal interval for Beagle dogs to at least ten minutes.

Comparing the different definitions we decided to define a "meal" as:

1. Total daily food sum: the total daily amount including every single amount that was eaten during the day, maximum of 450g (exceptions possible, depending on the body condition score of the individual dog)
2. Daily food intake of the meals: the single meals added together as the end sum of the day
3. Per single visit, the dog needs to eat at least 1g (average of half a pellet is 1.5g), food intake smaller than 1g are not counted as meals but make part of total daily food sum.
4. The minimum meal size for males is set to 10g, the one for females 8g. Meals smaller than 10g or 8g are not counted as meals will make part of total daily food sum.

5. The intermeal interval has to be longer than ten minutess from the end of the first food intake to the beginning of the food intake to separate two meals

The mean values of daily food intake (DFI) and single meals per visit, meal duration time (MDT) per day and also per single meal and the visits per day of all studies are analyzed. On days with no food intake, the parameters are set as zero, wrong data as described in 4.6.7 is not used for the calculation and the fields in the columns are left empty.

To determine the normal feeding behavior of dogs, the daily food intake (DFI), the meal duration time (MDT), and the number of visits per day (VpD), as well as the single meals and the single meal duration times of 459 dogs (227 females, 232 males) are recorded and evaluated. The studies are separated into the different study phases pretest, main phase and recovery for comparison. An abnormal feeding behavior is determined as a deviation from the normal values evaluated in the pretest. As for the determination of the MDT, only 448 animals are evaluated. Eleven animals had to be excluded due to wrong data as described in section 5.1.

For a better understanding of the meal definition, the single parameters are illustrated in an example in figure 4.10 to 4.12.

4.6.6 Use and function of FeeditManager

FeeditManager is the administrative Software of the automated dog feeder system.
The program permits feeding dogs in groups as well as performing studies based on feeding. Food amount and access to the feeder can be determined for all groups within a study or for each group and for each animal separately.

First select a study from the Feedit-Software. This could be an *actual*[a] study or a closed one, which could be found under *historical*[b].

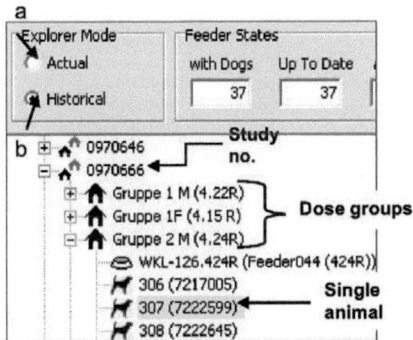

Figure 4.9: Selected study from the FeeditManager

By clicking on the plus "+" on the left side of the study number, the animals show up and the requested animal can be chosen.

Right hand click on the animal number opens the feeding activity of the chosen days.
All visits, even the ones with no food intake are listed as shown in figure 4.12. This interface is necessary for controlling the daily feeding activities of the dogs and the data in its propriety. Computerized analysis of presented results is not possible with this list, but can be summarized with another tab, which is described in 4.12.

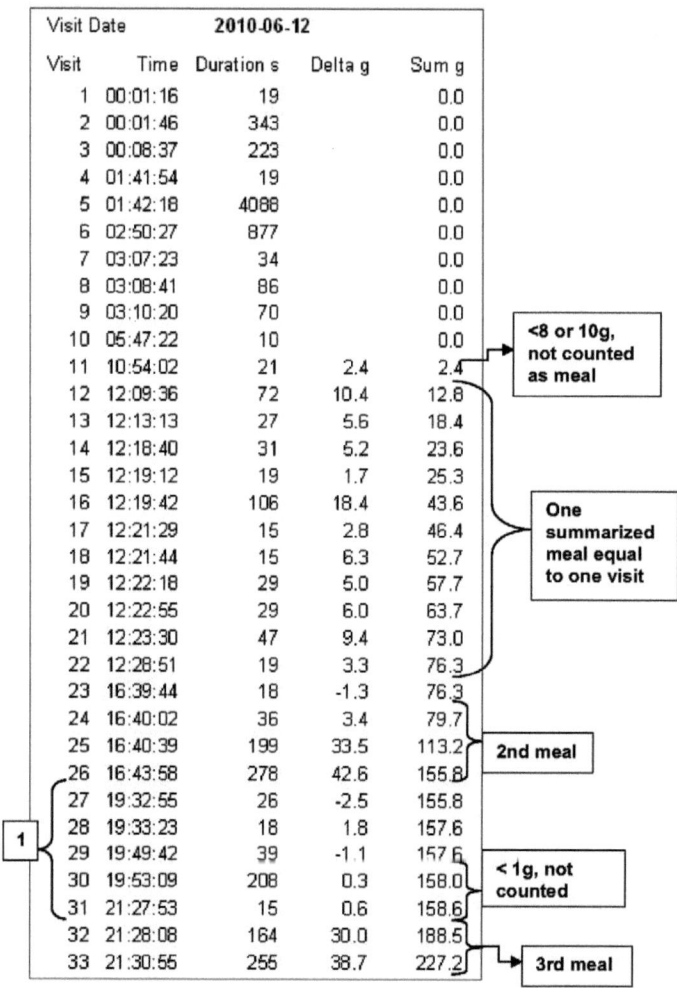

Figure 4.10: Illustration of the different parameter used for the meal definition: 1= *Intermeal interval*

Figure 4.10 illustrates the visits to the dog feeder including the time of day, the eaten amount of food and the time spent in the dog feeder. The dog in this example has already entered the dog feeder during the night. Due to the limited feeding hours from 10am to 11pm, the dog cannot eat until visit 11, when it ate 2.4g. No further food intake is recorded until 12pm and the amount is not included in the calculated meal sum as it is too small. From 12:09:36 to 12:28:51 the dog ate 73.9g. Due to the intermeal interval to the next food intake, which is longer than ten minutes, the 73.9g can be summarized as one meal. Two more meals are eaten during the day.

The summarized table of meals will open by clicking on a new tab.

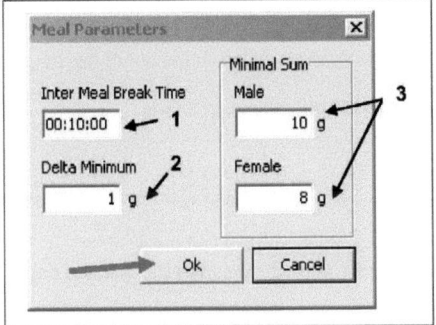

Figure 4.11: Window with the defined parameters: *1= Intermeal Interval, 2= minimum intake, 3= minimal total single meal amount*

When clicking "ok" (red arrow), the single visits and meals will be summarized into a list as shown below in figure 4.12 (the same animal from figure 4.10)

As the meal definition did not exist for food consumption analysis, it first had to be defined in a separate window in the software system and finally validated.

Visit Date	2010-06-12						
		1	5	2		3 Maximum Food per Day g	4 450
Visit	Time	Present s	Meal g	Rate g/s	Duration s	Meal Sum g	Sum g
1	12:09:36	409	73.9	0.180733	1174	73.9	76.3
2	16:40:02	513	79.5	0.154990	514	153.4	155.8
3	21:27:53	434	69.2	0.159544	437	222.7	227.2

Figure 4.12: Summarized visits into the defined meal: *1= entry time into the feeder, 2= amount/time, 3= Meal sum: total of counted meals, 4= Sum: Total of the daily intake with residuals smaller than the minimal meal amount; 5= single meal duration time in sec.*

Out of figure 4.12., the MDT (5) for each meal, the feed rate (2), the total daily food sum (4) and the DFI (3) are summarized. No. 1 points to the time of day, when the dog entered the dog feeder.
To serve as a good meal definition, the difference between total daily food intake and total meal sum should not be bigger than 10%.
(The summarized data can be saved into a CSV-Excel sheet and run through a Macro to tabulate the single parameters into columns.)

4.6.7 Errors occurring during feeding process

Errors occur in automated feeding machines. To minimize the number of errors in the data set, the values that may be wrong have first to be evaluated. The values that may be affected are single meals, single meal duration time and feeding rate. If these parameters are wrong, the DFI, MDT and VpD are incorrect as well.

The errors are either created by hardware or software problems.

Hardware or dog-dependent errors include:

- Unreal meal times due to dogs sleeping in the passage. The transponder receiver registers the dog and the doors stay open
- The doors do not close due to technical problems such as pellets in the door way, dogs cannot eat
- Doors do not open due to empty silo or empty food bowl, dogs cannot eat

Software errors:

- A meal duration time that is recorded as being too short due to signal problems with the transponder receiver
- Balance errors: incorrect value of the food left over due to wrong weighing
- Wrong measuring of the food intake, the measured amount exceeds 450g and the dog cannot eat anymore due to its limit of 450g
- Single food intake registered more than once

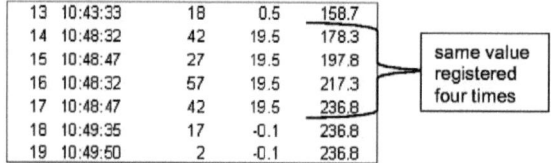

Figure 4.13: An error example: one meal measured four times

Various errors are already detected during the daily control of the hardware and software of the dog feeder, e.g. feeder errors or wrong amount of food intake.
Other errors such as dogs sleeping in the passage have to be first manually checked and identified prior to the analysis. Due to the large amount of data, the process is very time consuming.

4.7 Statistical Evaluation

The statistical evaluation is performed using the GNU R-statistical program
Linear mixed effect modeling – dog ID as the random effect, generalized additive models is used (advanced with random effects). Results are significant, if the p-value is > 0.05.
Excel Pivot and excel graphics for the charts of the feeding patterns are used.

5. Results

In the first part of this section an overview of the results of all dogs together will be given.

I will discuss three different feeding patterns with five examples that stood out in the analysis.

The dogs in group 4, in particular, will be looked at more closely, because their feeding behavior deviated most from the other groups.

Finally, the relationship between symptoms and food intake and general observations of the individual study phases will be presented.

5.1 General food intake behavior

Sixteen studies of the last four years were analyzed to evaluate the dogs' feeding behavior. The studies were chosen by several criteria as described in 4.2.1.
In general, a study contained 32 dogs. Three of the sixteen studies had fewer dosing groups, resulting in fewer dogs. All in all, 19 dogs had to be excluded for various reasons, e.g. early sacrifice or because they were manually fed and no data was available. There were fewer dogs left for the evaluation of the feeding patterns in the recovery phase. In total 60 males and 54 females from group 1 and 4 entered the recovery phase.
Females spent on average 21.6 mins to eat 270g per day. Males spent on average 19 mins to eat 329g. Both males and females made on average 3.7 visits per day.
In fifteen of the sixteen studies, male dogs ate significantly more than bitches ($p< 0.05$), but they also weighed 20% more than females. The average body weight of males was 9.9kg ± 0.7 and of females was 8.1kg ± 0.8. Food intake was 19% higher in males, correlating with the higher body weight.
In general, the dogs were allowed a maximum daily amount of 450g to eat from 10am to 11pm.
In three out of the sixteen studies, the limit of the daily amount of food was first set at 350g. The majority of the dogs from the three studies always ate their food allowance. After two weeks, about half way through the main study phase, the food allowance in two studies was increased to 450g due to loss of body weight in several dogs. In all other studies, food limit was set to 450g from the start of the pretest.

A few animals of the 459 dogs still lost body weight, even though they always ate their 450g. Hence their food allowance was raised to 650g.

There was considerable variation among individual animals in the frequency of feeder visits. The number ranged from zero to fourteen visits per day during the whole study period (pretest, main phase and recovery). Nevertheless, it can be said that most of the animals ate three to six times per day.
The ranges for DFI and MDT varied considerably, from zero to 450g (DFI) and from zero up to 50 mins (MDT). The variation in the DFI can be seen in the box plot of the next two charts.

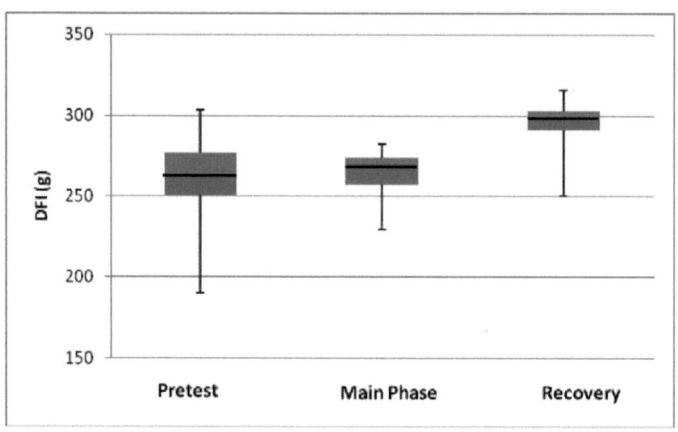

Chart 5.1: Box plot of the DFI of all females divided into the three study phases

The box plot demonstrates the variation of the values. The upper whisker marks the maximum value and the lower whisker the minimum value of the DFI. The black line in the box stands for the median and the upper and the lower border of the box are the 75% percentile and the 25% percentile, respectively.

The variation is most pronounced in the pretest, which can be seen by the long whiskers. This may assume that the female dogs ate more variably in the pretest compared to the other two study phases. This observation was not significantly evaluated.

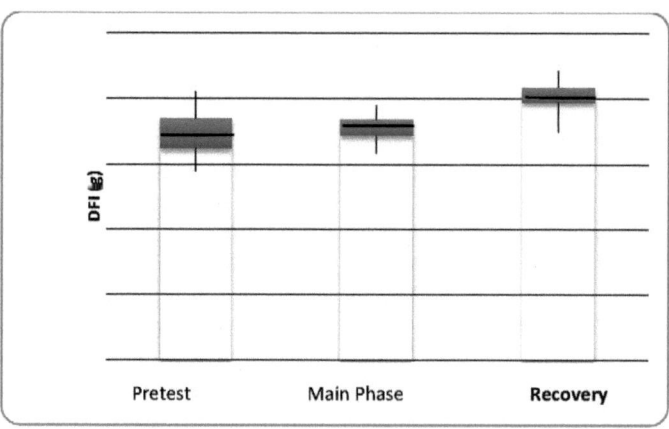

Chart 5.2: Box plot of the DFI of all males divided into the three study phases

The whiskers in chart 5.2 are short, which means that the values are in a closer range. The male dogs did not fluctuate from day to day that much.

The feeding patterns were evaluated in the pretest, the main phase and the recovery and were illustrated as the different parameters over time in line charts.

The statistical evaluation showed a significant decrease in food intake in ten out of the sixteen studies during the main phase compared to the pretest.
In two of the sixteen studies, a significant increase in food intake occurred during the main phase. In the remaining four studies, no significant correlation between dosing and food intake during the main phase was found.

The majority of the dogs (353 of 459 dogs) showed an irregular feeding behavior during the three study phases, which complicated the comparison and the interpretation of the different study phases. 84 dogs showed clear deviations of feeding behavior between the pretest and the main phase and 22 animals remained regular during the pretest and the main phase.
53 dogs had a constant pretest and main phase and 31 dogs were steady during the pretest, but became variable in the main phase.
Due to the lower number of dogs (only 114 animals) during recovery, this phase did not play such an important role as the pretest and the main phase. For that reason, I focused more on the deviations between the pretest and the main phase.

The MDTs should be considered with care from certain animals, in total from 45 dogs. They liked to sleep in the feeder after eating and their presence was erroneously recorded and added to the MDT, which affected the results. The evaluation of the meal duration time showed that dogs usually did not spend more than 1000s to eat a higher amount of food, e.g. 300g. For smaller amounts, the dogs usually spent on average between 150 and 300s.
Single meal duration times of values that seemed incorrect were compared with those that were correct and realistic within the study phase of the individual dog. In most cases, the amount eaten was low while the single meal duration time was too long, e.g. 900s for 15g.
The incorrect values were excluded and values from other single meal duration times of the same dog were chosen to replace the incorrect ones.
In cases where dogs slept in the feeder almost every day, results were noted as *not available (NA)* and no MDT was included in the statistical analysis.
Although the obviously wrong results from the 45 animals were corrected, some MDTs of a few animals could not be classified as either false or correct values. Considering the amount of data of 459 dogs, the values of the individual dogs were not considered to have significant influence on the overall results of the MDT.

As mentioned above, the dogs ate on average at least three to six times a day, split into one meal in the morning and one to two meals in the afternoon and evening. Various factors, e.g. the maximum plasma concentration (C_{max}) of the test substance may influence the time of the single meal intake during the day. In order to analyze for possible impacts on the single meals, the day was divided into four timeslots. The strongest impact on the animals' food intake was expected in the morning after administration. This is why the *early-slot* was chosen between 10am and 12pm. The other slots were divided in time intervals reasonably similar to each other.

Timeslots
- Early: meals between 10am and 12pm
- Afternoon: meals between 12pm and 16pm
- Evening: meals between 16pm and 20pm
- Late: meals between 20pm and 23pm

The intermeal intervals showed a clear break between the single meals which could be summarized into a daily sequence of the single meal intake during the day.
The morning meal was significantly measured as the biggest meal of the day. The other meal sizes eaten during the day became smaller from meal to meal. The meals late in the evening were usually more variable and small. Thus meals eaten in the later day time were less reliable due to variable sizes of the meals.

This made it more complicated to compare the timeslots of later daytimes, e.g. evening in the pretest with the evening-timeslots of the main phases. Hence, only morning meals were compared between the pretest and the main phase to detect any deviations.
In cases where dogs showed an inconsistent food intake in the morning, the single meals of the *early*-phase were inappropriate to compare between the different study phases.

In order to discuss the animals' feeding behavior more thoroughly, I added various tables and charts that allow looking at the results from different angles (females vs. males) and levels (whole study vs. group within study).

To start with an overview of the feeding behaviors' results, table 5.1 and 5.2 show the mean values of females and males in the three different study phases; pretest, main phase and recovery.

Table 5.1: Mean values of food intake of the females of all studies divided into the three study phases

All females (mean±SD)	Pretest	Main phase	Recovery
DFI (g)	262 ± 49	265 ± 70	292 ± 81
MDT(min)	19.7 ± 4.5	20.1 ± 5.9	23.2 ± 11.3
VpD	3.9 ± 0.9	3.7 ± 1	3.8 ± 1.3
Single meal (g)	62 ± 22	64 ± 23	72 ± 30
Single MDT (min)	4.9 ± 1.4	5.3 ± 3.7	5.6 ± 2.1

Legend: DFI= daily food intake, MDT= meal duration time, VpD= visits per day

The DFI of females was similar in the pretest and the main phase, but significantly increased in the recovery phase. The MDT only slightly non-significantly increased from the pretest to the main phase. From the main phase to the recovery, the MDT significantly increased. The number of VpD was similar in all three study phases.
The single meals from the pretest to the main phase was steady, while it significantly (p< 0.001) increased in the recovery from 62g (pretest) and 64g (main phase) to 72g. The dogs did not eat more often, which is seen in the steady number of VpD. As a consequence, they had to spend more time eating. The single meal duration time significantly slightly increased from 4.9mins to 5.3mins in the main phase and up to 5.6mins in the recovery.

Table 5.2: Mean values of food intake of the males of all studies divided into the three study phases

All Males (mean±SD)	Pretest	Main phase	Recovery
DFI (g)	332 ± 50.7	328 ± 79.3	352 ± 88.2
MDT (min)	18.6 ± 4.1	18.3 ± 5.6	20.2 ± 7.9
VpD	4 ± 1.1	3.7 ± 1.2	3.5 ± 1.4
Single meal (g)	74 ± 30	75 ± 26	88 ± 43
Single MDT (min)	4.2 ± 1.3	4.3 ± 1.7	5 ± 2.1

Legend: DFI= daily food intake, MDT= meal duration time, VpD= visits per day

The male dogs behaved similarly to the females. They had a significantly higher food intake in the recovery (352g) phase compared to the pretest (332g) and the main phase (328g). Unlike the females, the males' number of visits per day remained significantly lower in the recovery phase, while the MDT significantly slightly increased compared to the pretest and the main phase. The male dogs tended to eat faster with fewer visits with the same amount of food provided as in the pretest and main phase.

The tables 5.1 and 5.2 represent the total values for all groups together (controls and treated), however the different parameters for the dogs varied from group to group, which is illustrated as feeding patterns in chart 5.3 for females and in chart 5.4 for males.

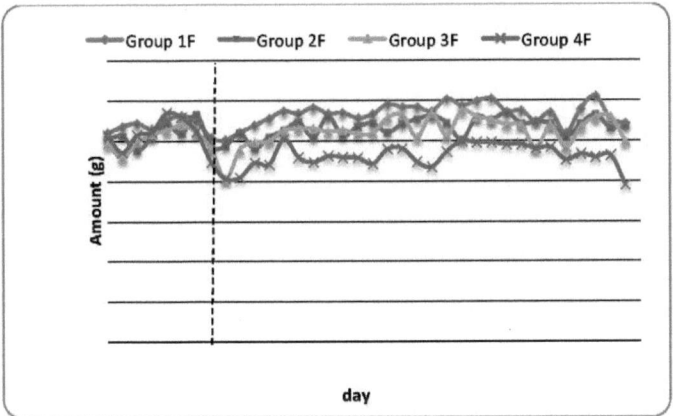

Chart 5.3: Average of DFI of all females divided into the four dose groups

During the pretest, the lines of all four groups run parallel to each other. On day 0, at the beginning of the main phase, a reduced food intake could be observed in all four female groups, most prominently in group 4 (violet) and only slightly in group 1 (blue). As mentioned in 4.5.2, the first three days led the dogs into a new situation. This may explain why they all ate less during the first three days.

Food intake of group 1 (blue) increased after the first days of the main phase while group 2 (red) and 3 (green) remained steady. Group 4 (violet) had the lowest food intake. Possible reasons for this feeding pattern will be explained in section 5.2 where particular examples are analyzed in more detail.

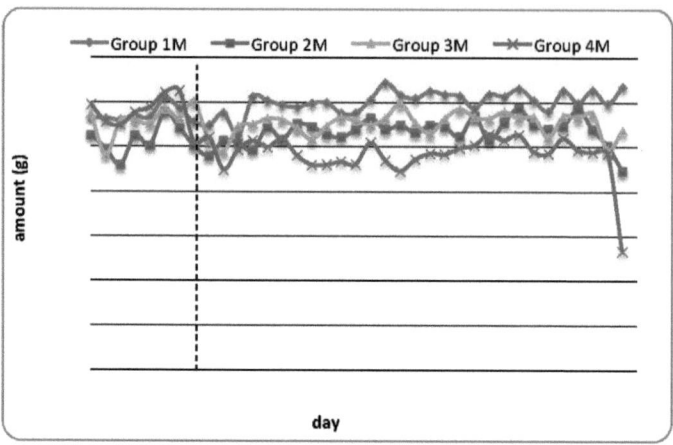

Chart 5.4: Average of DFI of males divided into the four dose groups

As mentioned earlier males generally ate more than females. Nevertheless, the feeding pattern of males looks similar to the feeding pattern of females. The males also reacted at day 0 with a lower food intake, but not as strongly as the females. The diagram of chart 5.4 containing all four male groups shows an increase in food intake in group 1 (blue) and a decrease in group 4 (violet) as already seen in females in chart 5.3.

Chart 5.3 and 5.4 show clearly that the dosage had a similar effect on both sexes. The male control group (group 1) as well as the female control group (group 1) had a significant higher food intake than the high dose groups (group 4) of both sexes. Thus, it can be said so far that the test substances may have an effect on both sexes and their feeding patterns. This is shown by the lower food intake lines (violet) in the diagram of chart 5.3 (females) and chart 5.4 (males).

For completeness I have added charts 5.5 (females) and 5.6 (males). They illustrate the MDTs of the different dose groups of both sexes. The plots in chart 5.5 and 5.6 run in similar manner to those of chart 5.3 and 5.4. This means that MDTs correlate with the amount of the DFI.

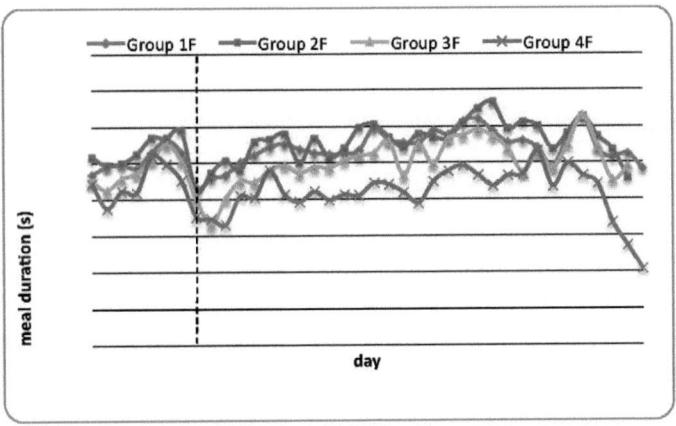

Chart 5.5: Average of the daily MDT of all females divided into the four dose groups

Just like in chart 5.3 and 5.4, it can be seen that females reacted stronger than males on day 0. Group 4 was lower than the others, correlating with the lower food intake of female group 4 in chart 5.3. This was not the case with males. Male group 4 did not have a clearly shorter MDT as the other groups, although this group had a lower food intake as well.

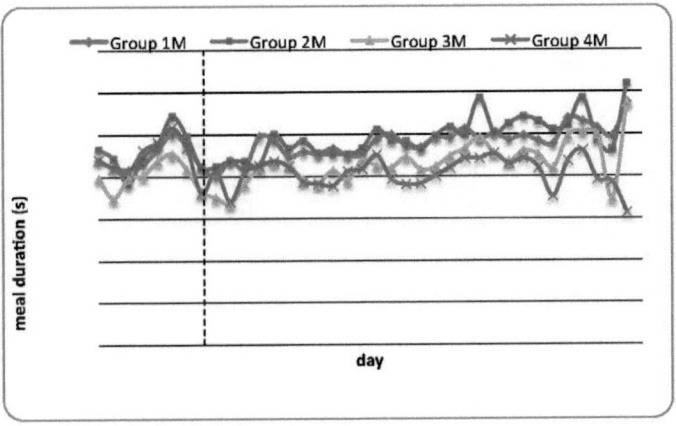

Chart 5.6: Average of the daily MDT of all males divided into the four dose groups

Due to the deviations found in the feeding behavior of both groups 4 (females and males), as seen in chart 5.3 and 5.4, I considered it necessary to look at them more closely. Hence, the individual mean values of group 4 of both sexes are shown in table 5.3 (females) and 5.4 (males). The mean values of the other groups are listed in the appendix.

Table 5.3: Mean values of all females in group 4 divided into the three study phases

Group 4F (mean±SD)	Pretest	Main phase	Recovery
DFI (g)	256 ± 50.6	229 ± 86	278 ± 93
MDT (min)	17.1 ± 3.4	17.4 ± 5.8	24.1 ± 14
VpD	3.7 ± 0.2	3.3 ± 0.3	3.9 ± 1.2
Single meal (g)	62 ± 22	61 ± 24	66 ± 22.4
Single MDT (min)	4.6 ± 1.3	5.4 ± 1.4	5.4 ± 2.1

Legend: DFI= daily food intake, MDT= meal duration time, VpD= visits per day

During the pretest, females ate a daily amount of 256g in 17.1 mins and 3.7 visits. In the main phase, the DFI as well as the number of VpD was significantly lower, but the MDT remained steady. It can be seen that the amount of single meals remained steady from the pretest to the main phase. The single meal duration time, however, significantly increased from 4.6 mins in the pretest to 5.4 mins in the main phase.

It can be assumed that the female dogs needed more time to eat the same amount or even a smaller amount of food in the main phase compared to the pretest. It is possible that they ate slower due to a reduced wellbeing.

In the recovery phase, however, the DFI as well as the MDT significantly increased compared to the main phase. The MDT increased from 17.4 mins to 24.1 mins. Additionally the DFI was 20g higher in the recovery phase. A positive correlation between DFI and MDT was restored.

Table 5.4: Mean values of all males in group 4 divided into the three study phases

Group 4M (mean±SD)	Pretest	Main phase	Recovery
DFI (g)	339 ± 43	295 ± 97	333 ± 101
MDT (min)	16.7 ± 3	19.4 ± 6.2	20.5 ± 9.9
VpD	3.9 ± 0.2	3.4 ± 0.2	3.5 ± 0.3
Single meal	78 ± 29	69 ± 33	84 ± 36
Single MDT (min)	4.6 ± 1.2	4.3 ± 1.5	5 ± 1.8

Legend: DFI= daily food intake, MDT= meal duration time, VpD= visits per day

Male dogs showed a similar feeding behavior compared to the females. They also had a significant lower DFI (295g) in the main phase compared to the pretest (339g). The amount of the single meals became non-significant smaller while the meal duration time of the single meals remained steady. Similar to the females, the male dogs needed more time to eat a smaller amount of food in the main phase.

No changes in MDT were measured during the recovery phase compared to the main phase. The steady MDT and VpD but an increased DFI during the recovery imply that the dogs must have eaten faster. The single meals and the single MDT were significantly smaller in the main phase compared to the recovery phase.

Looking at the results of tables 5.1-5.4, it can be said that females and males both ate more during the recovery phase than in the main phase. But while females needed more time to eat the larger amount of food, males ate faster.

In 47 of the 114 animals that entered the recovery phase, the DFI in the recovery phase was higher than in the main phase. The opposite was observed in only fourteen animals. The other animals had an equal food intake in the main phase and the recovery phase.
The results of the comparison between the DFI of the pretest with the recovery looks similar. 40 dogs had a higher food intake in the recovery compared to the pretest and 26 animals had a lower food intake in the recovery compared to the pretest. In 32 animals, food intake was equal between the two study phases.

Eight animals from two studies had to be excluded due to different food allowance. During the pretest and the first two weeks of the main phase, the dogs had a food allowance of 350g. They ate more when food allowance was raised to 450g after the first two weeks of the main phase, resulting in higher DFI. Due to the variance of the two food allowances, the data of the DFI could not be compared between the three study phases.

5.1.1 Body weight
In studies with no impact on food intake, no effect was measured on the dogs' body weight. Nevertheless, a loss in body weight appeared as expected in studies with a negative impact on food intake. Certain animals including control animals lost body weight within the four study weeks of the main phase, even though no change in food consumption was measured. On some occasions, the dogs ate even more from week to week and still lost body weight. The increased energy intake may be due to stress caused by the study conduct and the test substance's effect.
Body weight was only taken once to twice weekly and no daily comparisons were possible.

5.2. Three feeding patterns and their examples
Throughout the sixteen studies, the dogs reacted with various feeding patterns. In order to enable a structured discussion of the results, the feeding behaviors were classified into the following three feeding patterns:

- No impact: there was no change observed in the whole study

- Irregular impact: Some animals of one group showed a reaction by an increased or decreased food intake during the study, others did not

- Strong impact: A change in feeding behavior shown by decreased or increased food intake could be observed in all animals of the same dose group

Throughout the sixteen studies, the reaction of one dog could occasionally deviate from another dog's reaction within the same group. This means, for example, that a dog could show a delayed reaction or no reaction at all, while the other dogs showed a clear impact. Thus, certain animals' behavior was contradictory to the general feeding pattern of the group. The accumulation of the test substance in the dog's plasma may be one explanation, but was not further analyzed.

As the presentation of the results of all sixteen studies (459 dogs) exceeds the scope of this work, I have chosen five of the sixteen studies that serve as representative examples for the three feeding patterns stated above. All five examples were performed under the same conditions (pretest, main phase and recovery) and contained four dose groups with group 1 as the control group and group 4 as the high dose group.

Study A illustrates the feeding pattern with no obvious impact on the feeding behavior. In Study B the feeding pattern with an irregular impact on the feeding behavior will be shown. In this example, two different reactions of the irregular feeding behavior can be demonstrated. As the *strong* impact feeding pattern showed various reactions, I have chosen three examples (Study C, D and E) to demonstrate this feeding pattern. Study C and D describe the situation of an immediate strong impact (Study C) and a delayed strong impact (Study D) on the feeding behavior. The last example, Study E will illustrate a reaction of increased food intake.

Deviations to the feeding behavior occurred most often in group 4 and less often in groups with lower dose (group 2 and 3). That is, why in the examples presented, mostly group 4 and group 1 only are discussed. Group 1 was administered with a placebo and no drug-induced reactions were expected. This group served as the reference group and could be compared with the other groups that showed deviations of the feeding patterns. Nevertheless, reactions that were not associated to the test substance were observed in the control group.

5.2.1 First example: Study A with no Impact

The first example is a study with slight or no relevant changes of the feeding behavior. If deviations of the feeding pattern occurred, no correlation to the treatment with the test substance could be found. As mentioned earlier, the food intake could vary from day to day, which can be seen in the charts in this example. The fluctuation of the DFI made it difficult to interpret the results and to make a clear statement about the cause of the variable feeding pattern.

The following chart outlines the averages of the female dogs' feeding behavior. The individual lines represent the different dose groups.

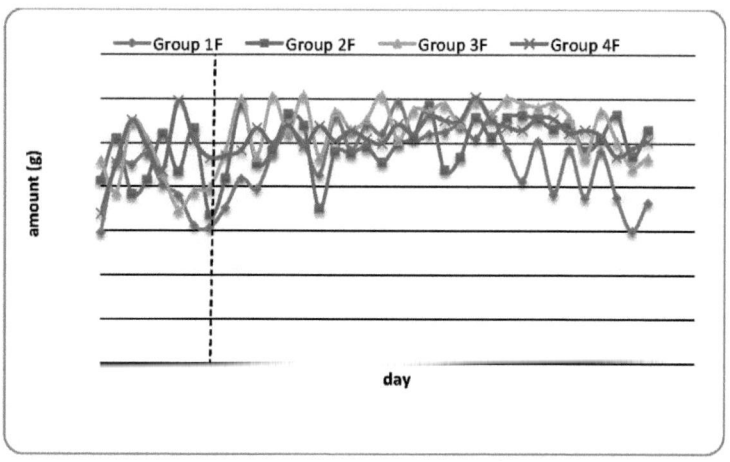

Chart 5.7: Average of DFI of females of study A

In chart 5.7, females of group 1 (blue) started to reduce their DFI on day -3, lasting until day 0. From day 1 on the food intake increased again.
Thus, the reduced food intake could not be associated with the influence of the test substance or with the beginning of the administrations in the main phase, because it started before the test substance was dosed.
Group 2 (red) seemed more regular during the pretest than group 1, but also had a lower food intake on day 0. In cases with an impact on the food intake that starts on day 0 of the main phase, the analyzing of the DFI should not only include the average DFI of the group, but also the DFI of the individual dogs.
Group 3 (green) had a fluctuating food intake during the pretest, which increased from study day -1 on. The dosing and the in-life examinations did not start before day 0, hence it can be assumed that the dogs were not distracted from their feeding pattern at the beginning of the main phase.

While the pretest of group 4 was variable, the main phase became constant and slightly increased until the end of the main phase. No drug-induced effect could be observed.
All four groups ate within a range of 250 to 330g per day during the pretest and 300 to 350g in the main phase with a few outliers. Due to these results, it can be assumed that the animals were not affected by the test substance and were in good health.

Female group 4 is shown separately for a better illustration of the different reactions of the dogs with the highest dose.

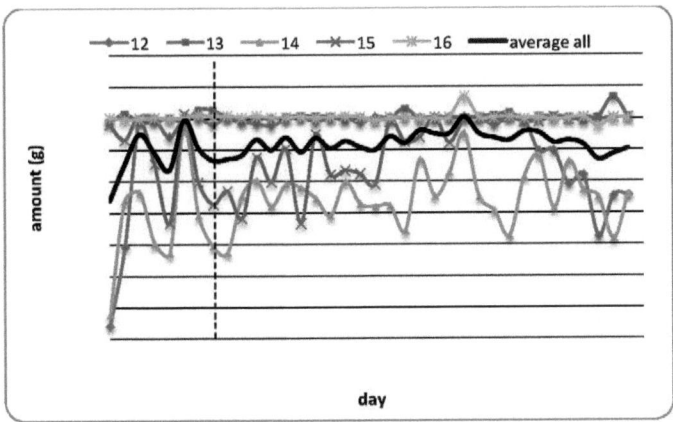

Chart 5.8: Average of DFI of female group 4

When taking a closer look at the single animals of female group 4, it is noticeable that three animals (12, 13, 16) had a very steady food intake and ate their daily food allowance of 350g. Animal no. 14 had an irregular food intake during the pretest, but became more regular in the main phase. Dog no. 15 was variable during the pretest and the main and an interpretation of its feeding behavior is not possible.
The black line represents the average DFI of group 4. Food intake in the main phase was more regular than in the pretest. Nevertheless, the dogs had a short period of lower food intake within the first three days of the main phase.

All parameters (e.g. DFI, MDT, VpD) first have to be analyzed before it can be said that the animals were not distracted from eating. One parameter alone is not as meaningful. The effects on VpD and MDT are explained later in chart 5.10.

The single dogs of male group 4 did not have to be presented separately, because the line of the food intake of chart 5.9 reflects the feeding pattern of all male dogs.

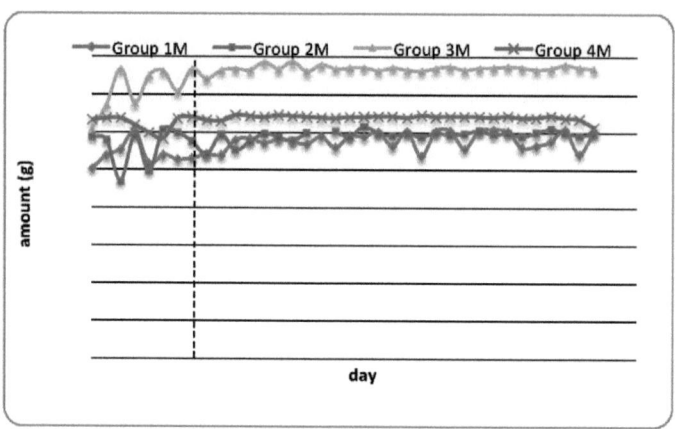

Chart 5.9: Average of DFI of males of study A

Male dogs had a steady food intake as shown in chart 5.9, independent of the dose group and study phase. They did not show any reaction at the beginning of the main phase (dashed line). Group 3 had a higher food intake due to a higher limit of daily food amount of one dog. As mentioned earlier, certain dogs had a higher energy requirement due to their body condition. Consequently, the food intake in group 3 was also significantly higher ($p<0.05$), but not reliable due to different limits of food. The DFI of all male dogs was not influenced by the start of the administrations and the in-life examinations that started on day 0.

Even though, the daily food intake of males of study A did not show any deviations from the normal DFI, this does not mean that no reactions could be observed. Deviations of the VpD and the MDT may have been observed.

In certain cases, the VpD and the DFI were variable at the beginning of a new phase and became both steady when the dog adapted to the new daily routine. In other cases, only the VpD was variable, while DFI remained constant. Both reactions illustrated a deviation from the normal feeding behavior. The influence on the VpD can be observed in chart 5.10.

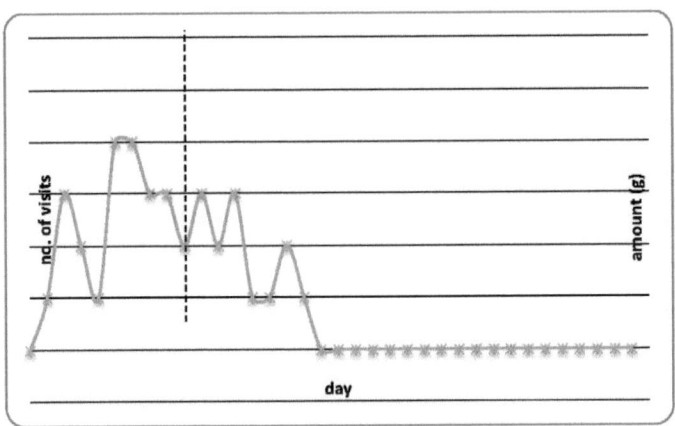

Chart 5.10: DFI and VpD of one dog out of male group 1

The dog of male group 1 in chart 5.10 had a high and variable number of VpD during the pretest and the first week of the main phase, even though food intake was steady with only one outlier on day -3. The number of visits decreased and became steady after the first week. Situations like this with a decrease of visits after a few days, was observed in the majority of dogs. Normally, the lower number of visits went hand in hand with the beginning of constant food consumption. Sometimes variable food intake still persisted, while the Vpd stayed in a steady range. A decreased number of visits with an increased or steady DFI was observed in 36 dogs (7.8%).

Eating the whole 350g at a time as seen in chart 5.10 was rarely observed. Normally the dogs split the daily amount in at least two meals per day.

Body weight in all four dose groups of both sexes remained steady or increased slightly.

5.2.2 Second example: Study B with irregular impact

In study B, I want to demonstrate the impact on food intake at the beginning of the main phase with a recovering period after the first week. The situation was only observed in part of female group 4. Males did not show a clear reaction on food intake that could have been associated to the test substance.

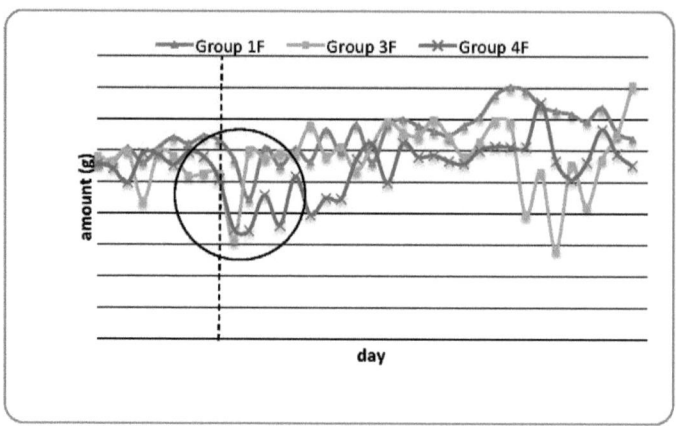

Chart 5.11: Average of DFI of female group 1,3,and 4

For a better overview, group 2 was left out in chart 5.11 (no impact was seen in this group). The black circle in chart 5.11 marks the decreased food intake of group 3 (green) and 4 (violet). Group 3 had a lower food intake only on the second day while food intake of group 4 decreased as well on the second day, but recovered within the subsequent week.
The daily amount of food was set at 450g instead of 350g after two weeks of the main phase. As mentioned earlier, this was done based on the higher required energy intake of the dogs. The DFI, especially the one of group 3, were quite variable during the last week of the main phase. Possbily that the dogs first had to get used to the new limit of food allowance and their food intake became irregular until they had adapted to it. This reaction was observed in 16 dogs of the 62 dogs that were affected by the raise of food allowance. 12 dogs remained stable and 34 dogs were variable during the whole time of the main phase, independent of the food allowance.
Due to the higher food intake from day 17 onwards, only food intake until day 16 was included in the evaluation of mean values particularly for this example.
The mean values of the DFI of the recovery phase were not compared with those of the main phase due to the two different limits of food allowance.

A significantly lower food intake ($p<0.05$) in group 4 in the main phase was evaluated, correlating with the lower food intake of the females at the beginning of the main phase.

In order to show the lower food intake of female group 4, a separate chart of this group was added.

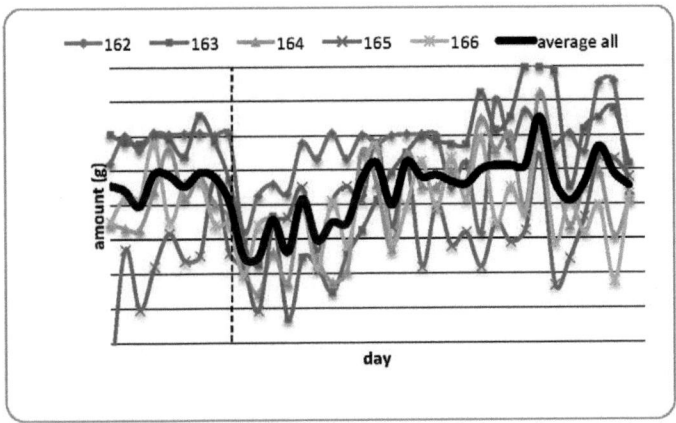

Chart 5.12: Average of DFI of female group 4 of study B

Animal no. 1=blue, no. 2=red, no.3=green, no. 4=violet, no. 5=orange

No. 162 (blue), 163 (red) and 164 (green) are good examples of a deviation of the regular feeding pattern. The dogs had a fairly steady food consumption during the pretest except for dog no. 164 that was more variable in the pretest. From day 0 on, the food intake decreased to almost half of the amount in the pretest. During the main phase, the DFI slowly increased again, but remained irregular.

Dogs no. 165 (violet) and 166 (orange) were not that clear to interpret. Food intake of both dogs was variable. Dog no. 165 had only on day 2 a clear lower food intake compared to the rest of the days, while dog no. 166 had a lower food intake on day 1. One day of low food intake could not be associated to the drug-induced effect and could be caused by various reasons.

This study is also a good example to demonstrate the impact not only on the DFI. The sequence of the single meals during the day changed. The day times of the consumed meals in the pretest were compared with the ones in the main phase which enabled me to detect whether the meals had shifted or not. An overview of the single meals is given in chart 5.13.

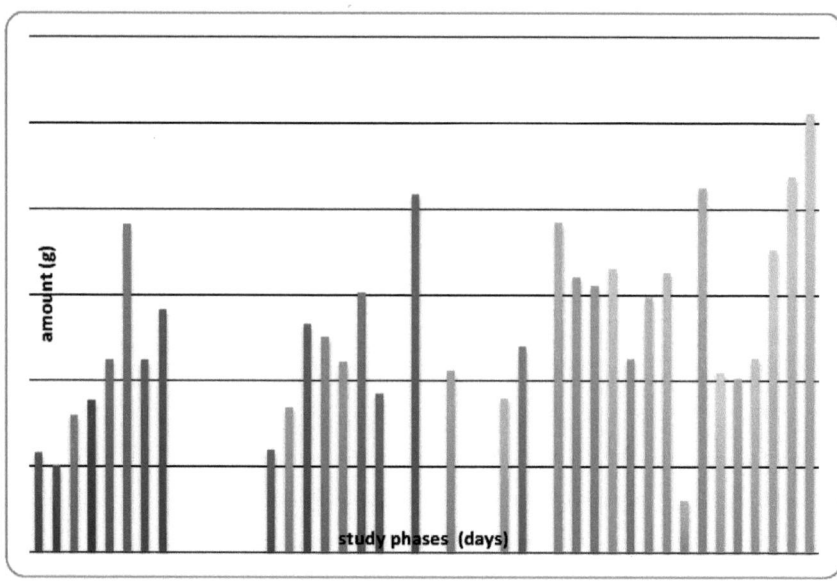

Chart 5.13: Average of the single meals of one dog of female group 4 of study B, divided into the timeslots

In chart 5.13 the pretest (day-7 to -1) was compared with the first week of the main phase (day 0 to day7). Three timeslots are presented, but only the one of *1 early* showed a clear deviation in the main phase when compared to the pretest. The timeslot *late* was left out; it was not relevant in this study example.

During the pretest, this dog in chart 5.13 ate at least once in the morning every day, but skipped the morning meals and occasionally left out the afternoon meals from day 1 to day 5. The single meals in the *evening* remained steady.

The *early* timeslot is illustrated separately in chart 5.14 which enabled a close comparison between the pretest and the whole main phase.

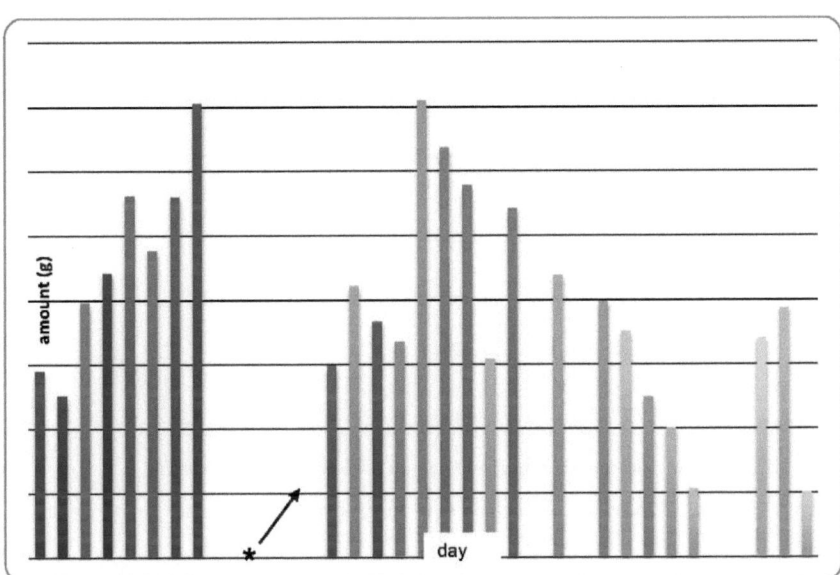

Chart 5.14: Average of the single meals of the same dog as in chart 5.13, only the early phase;
* = the break between day 0 and day 6 with no food intake

Due to the non-significant deviations that were seen in the early phase chart 5.14 concentrates on this phase only. The whole female group reacted more or less in a similar way during this phase. Thus, this particular dog may stand for the whole group. During the pretest, the dog ate every day in the morning, but left out morning meals during the main phase.

The star marks the period of days with no food intake in the morning. The dog started to eat again in the morning from day 6 onwards. At the end of the main phase, the dog did not eat on day 23 and 24. A probable reason for this may have been the in-life examinations that were performed on these days that distracted the dog from its normal feeding pattern.

When analyzing the feeding pattern of the DFI in chart 5.12 in combination with the single meal pattern, a non-significant deviation of the feeding behavior could also be observed for dog no. 165 and 166. They had more or less similar mean values of the DFI in the pretest and the main phase, but left out the single meals in the morning.

This reaction of skipped or lower single meals was not only seen in this female high dose group (group 4). Animals of other studies and other group belonging also showed deviations from the normal feeding pattern during the first days of the main phase by skipping their meals. In cases of control animals (group 1) the morning meals usually were not left out, but the amount of food eaten was lower within the first two to four days than on other days, possibly due to the stressful time within the first three days. These observations were not statistically analyzed and no significance is available.

Furthermore it was observed that dogs that skip the morning meals started to eat more frequently in the *evening-* and *late*-phase.

Contrary to the females of group 4, males did not show a visible impact on DFI at the beginning of the main phase, which is illustrated in chart 5.15.

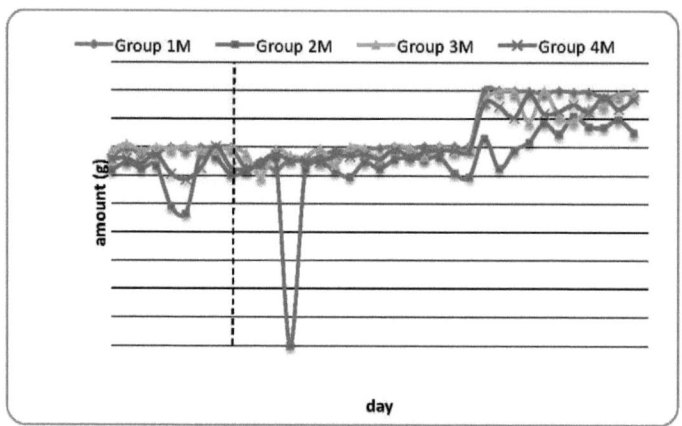

Chart 5.15: Average daily food intake of male group 1-4 from the example study

Chart 5.15 shows all male groups of study B. In the pretest and in the main phase, small fluctuations appeared, but a clear reaction could not be observed.
Male group 4 (violet) was steady and the dogs ate as much as the dogs of control group 1 (blue). Further analyzing of the toxicokinetic results may have been worth to evaluate a possible explanation for the different reactions on food intake between males and females of the high dose group of this study.

As shown in chart 5.15, dogs of male group 4 did not show a reaction at the beginning of the main phase, when the dosing started. They also ate more when food limit was raised from 350g to 450g. Noteworthy was the comparison of the recovery phase with the main phase of this group. I have chosen two dogs that I will discuss more closely in the following two charts. They showed an interesting change in food intake in the recovery phase.

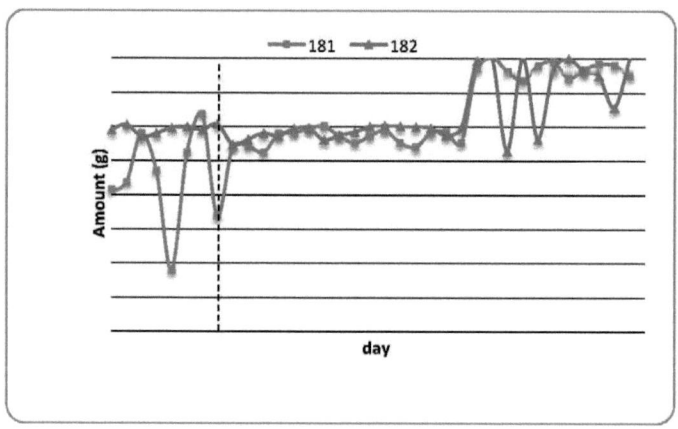

Chart 5.16: DFI during pretest and main phase of the two dogs of male group 4

In chart 5.16, the food intake of the two dogs during the pretest and main phase is illustrated. Dog 181 had a variable food intake during the pretest, but became steady from day 1 onwards of the main phase. Dog 182 (red line) was steady from the beginning of the pretest until the daily food limit was raised to 450g. Between day 19 and 21 food intake was variable, but became steady again as soon as the dog was used to the higher limit of daily food intake. Focusing only on the DFI (VpD and MDT not included), the drug administration and the examinations had no influence on the dogs' eating behavior.

Continuing into the recovery phase of these two dogs of male group 4, a clear effect could be seen in chart 5.17.

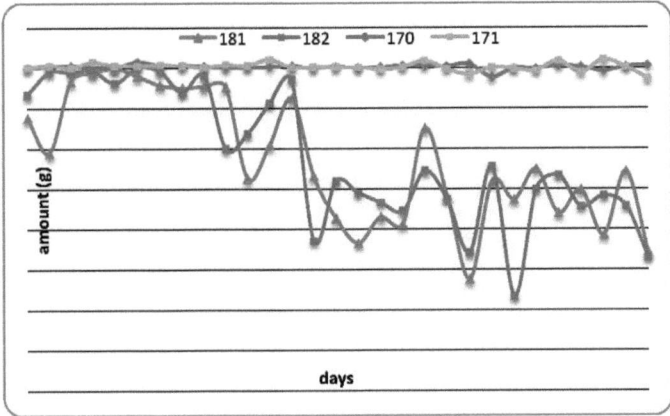

Chart 5.17: DFI during the recovery phase of the two dogs of male group 4

The dogs still had a steady food intake during the first week of the recovery phase. Nevertheless, from day 10 until day 14, food intake decreased slowly. From day 14 onwards, the food intake of the two dogs remained within a range of 200 and 300g per day.

Only assumptions could be made why the dogs ate less in the recovery. The lower food intake may be caused by a lower need of energy intake. Dogs are capable of controlling their energy intake by eating more or less calories.
In the recovery phase, the dogs may have been less active due to the smaller number of animals. Other possible reasons for a lower required energy intake may have been the calmer environment due to no examinations or no drug-induced effect.

This explanation that lower food intake may be due to a reduced need of energy intake became more likely, when the daily food intake and body weight of group 4 with the control group (dog no. 170 and 171) were compared during the main phase and the recovery phase.

The DFI in the recovery phase of male group 1 was steady in contrary to the one of male group 4, which could be seen in chart 5.17.

The two dogs of male group 1 had a steady food intake during the main phase and recovery phase. The lines of the food intake of group 1 were already illustrated in chart 5.15, thus only the recovery phase of the two male dogs were visualized in chart 5.17. The DFI of both animals was very constant throughout the whole recovery phase. The feeding behavior of both dogs was neither influenced in the main phase nor in the recovery phase. This lets us conclude that the animals were not distracted by the in-life examination or the administration.

Body weight

The dogs of male group 1 had an initial body weight of 9.5kg. At the end of the main phase, their body weight dropped to 8.8kg, even though, they always ate their entire daily food

allowance, as seen in chart 5.15. During the recovery phase, the body weight increased again to 9.4kg. It would have been interesting to see, whether they would have started to eat less or not after reaching their initial body weight.
Male group 4 gained body weight during the study while the other male groups lost body weight.
The initial body weight of the two dogs of male group 4 was 8.9kg and 7.6kg, respectively. The body weight of both animals stayed steady during the main phase. In the recovery phase, they started to gain weight within the first week. This may explain the reduced food intake after the first week of the recovery phase. At the end of the recovery phase, they weighed 9.3kg and 8.1kg, respectively.

Two females of group 3 lost almost 1kg of body weight during the main phase. The females of group 4 also lost body weight, but regained most of it at the end of the main phase. The two females that entered the recovery phase did not lose body weight. Those were the two animals (no. 164 and 165) that did not show a clear reaction on food intake in chart 5.12. Their body weight correlated with the food intake that was not lower than in the pretest.

5.2.3 Third example: Study C with a clear impact at the beginning of the dosing part of both sexes

In this example, an impact on all dogs (males and females) of group 4 at the beginning of the main phase could be seen. Only some dogs partly recovered back to a normal feeding behavior. The dogs ate significantly less in the main phase compared to the pretest. Reasons for this will be explained in the following charts.

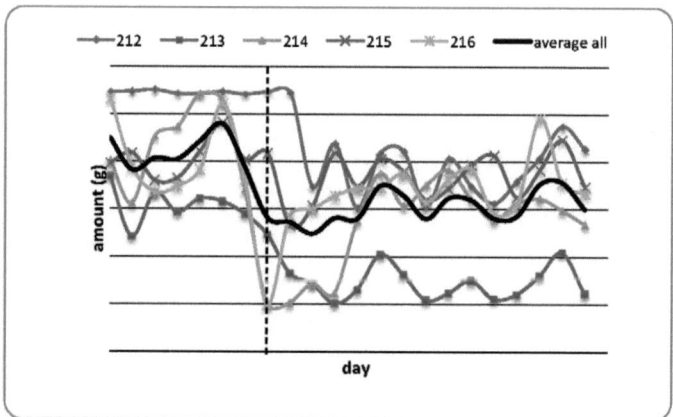

Chart 5.18: Average DFI of female group 4 of study C

In chart 5.18, the five dogs of female group 4 showed a deviation from the normal feeding behavior. This manifested itself in different feeding behaviors that all began from day 0 onwards of the main phase except for animal no. 212, which did not show a reaction before day 2.

Dog no. 212 (blue), 213 (red), 214 (green) and 216(orange) all reacted with a lower food intake either during the whole main phase or at least during the first week of the main phase.

The impact on food intake could also be expressed with the average DFI of all five dogs (black line). The DFI of the group was clearly lower in the main phase compared to the pretest.

Only dog no. 215 (violet) did not show a clear reaction on its feeding pattern. The dog ate variably during the pretest and the main phase and the level of the food intake stayed within a constant range of 200 and 300g.

Chart 5.19 illustrates the male dogs' feeding behavior. A clear deviation of the feeding behavior of male dogs could be seen.

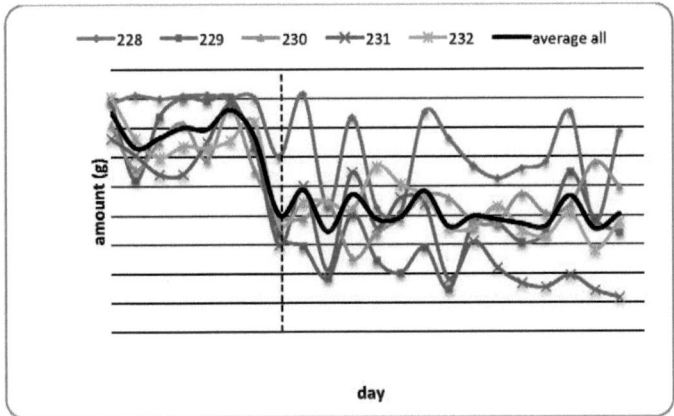

Chart 5.19: Average DFI of male group 4 of study C

The male dogs ate more regularly during the pretest than the females. They also ate less from day 0 when compared to females. Food intake was lower during the main phase than during the pretest.

As all five female and male dogs showed an impact on food intake in the main phase, it was concluded that it was drug-induced. Furthermore, the lower food intake in group 4 of both sexes was significantly lower ($p < 0.0001$) compared to the other dose groups.

If the impact on food intake was so strong, other parameters do not necessarily have to be evaluated. In other words, the other parameters, such as VpD or MDT are particularly helpful if the impact on food intake is not that clear or if only single animals of one group react.

Nevertheless, it was still worthwhile examining how the other parameters changed, if the feeding pattern was influenced. This is demonstrated in charts 5.19 and 5.20.

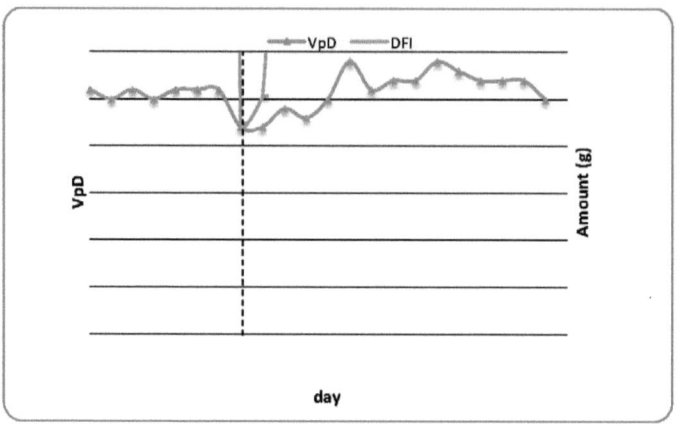

Chart 5.20: Average DFI and VpD of one female of group 4 of study C

The female dog in chart 5.20 ate less during the first two days of the pretest. After the first two days, the amount of food increased, but the number of visits remained steady. This was interpreted as a reaction of adaption to the new situation and as a sign of being in good health.

However, on day 0, no food intake was measured. The food intake increased gradually after the first two days of the main phase. After the first week of the main phase, the dog ate a little more than half of what it ate during the pretest. Further, the number of visits in the main phase was almost twice as high compared to the pretest phase. It is assumed that due to an effect of the test substance the dog did not feel well, resulting in smaller amounts split in several visits. This reaction was observed in 28 dogs (6.1%).

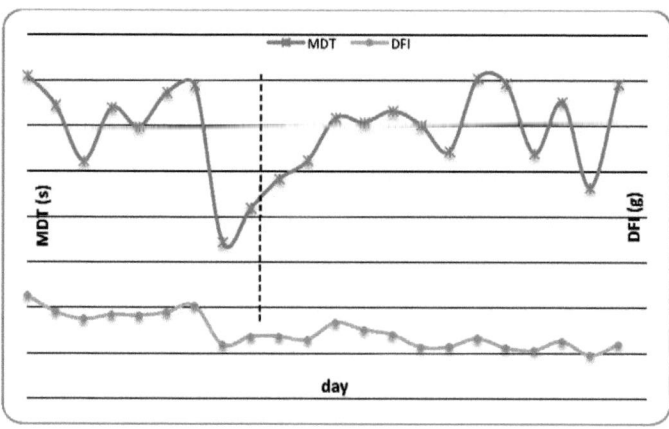

Chart 5.21: DFI and MDT of one male dog of high dose group 4

In chart 5.21, the same effect on the MDT as described in chart 5.20 for the VpD was observed. While the DFI decreased, the MDT increased, resulting in smaller, but longer meals.

A prolonged MDT while the size of the DFI became smaller could be observed in 16 dogs (3.5%) that showed a reaction on the feeding pattern.

Body weight

Males of group 1-3 gained weight or their body weight remained constant while group 4 lost over 1.5 kg of body weight (10.8kg in the pretest to 9.2kg at the end of the main phase) until the end of the main phase.

Females of group 1-3 only lost between 300 and 500g of body weight by the end of the main phase, while group 4 lost over 1kg.
The clear loss of body weight of both sexes in group 4 correlated with the low food intake, most likely reflecting a reduced wellbeing of these animals.

5.2.4 Fourth example: Study D with a clear impact, not only in high dose groups

The delayed effect of a test substance in this study did not only appear in the high dose groups (group 4) of both sexes, but also in the low dose female group 2 and in the middle dose group 3 of both sexes.

In this example, the correlation of the appearance of clinical symptoms with the changes in the feeding patterns will also be discussed.

The different reactions in the low dose group 2 of both sexes are presented in chart 5.22 for females and 5.23 for males.

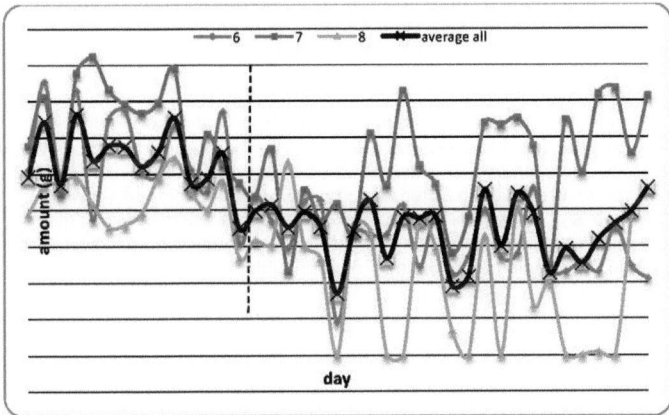

Chart 5.22: Average DFI of female group 2

The feeding pattern of female group 2 changed after the first three days of the main phase. Food intake of all three animals decreased, which is illustrated by the black line (average all). Animal no. 7 was not as strongly affected as the other two dogs (no. 6 and 8).

The test substance more than likely had an effect on the feeding pattern of female group 2, but no such reaction was seen in male group 2. Before continuing with male group 2 in chart 5.23, table 5.5 lists the symptoms that were observed in females group 2. Table 5.5 enables a comparison between the symptoms and the DFI. The comparison between the DFI and the observed symptoms may be helpful to explain a deviation of the normal feeding behavior of the particular dogs.

Table 5.5: Symptoms of two female dogs of the low dose group (Group 2)

Animal no.	Sign Type	Sign	Modifier	First day	Last day	Duration (days)
6	NORMAL	No remarkable clinical observations		1	18	18
	NEUROMUSCULAR	Wet-dog shakes		12	12	1
	EYES	Dried material around	Directional: both	19	30	12
	LIMBS	Limping	Limb: forelimb, right	29	30	2
7	NORMAL	No remarkable clinical observations		1	13	13
	EYES	Discharge	Directional: both	8	8	1
	GENERAL BEHAVIOR	Trembling		8	8	1
	GENERAL BEHAVIOR	Licking excessively		8	9	2
	NEUROMUSCULAR	Motor activity decreased	Grade: slight	8	11	4
	GENERAL BEHAVIOR	Trembling		11	11	1
	NEUROMUSCULAR	Motor activity decreased	Grade: marked	13	13	1
	GENERAL BEHAVIOR	Trembling		13	14	2
	NEUROMUSCULAR	Motor activity decreased	Grade: slight	14	16	3
	NORMAL	No remarkable clinical observations		15	22	8
	GENERAL BEHAVIOR	Trembling		17	17	1
	EYES	Dried material around	Directional: right	23	24	2
	NORMAL	No remarkable clinical observations		25	26	2
	SKIN/FUR	Staining	Location: back	27	30	4

Each symptom was recorded separately. The column "first day" refers to the first day during the study, i.e. the day of the main phase that the symptom first appeared. The symptoms could last for a few days. Thus, the "last day" column refers to the day that a symptom was observed for the last time. The total duration of the symptoms are listed in the last column.

Except for the symptom of dried material under the eyes, dogs no. 6 (blue line in chart 5.22) and 8 (green line in chart 5.22) did not show any relevant symptoms, which could have had an effect on food intake.

Dog no. 7 (red line in chart 5.22) developed various neuromuscular and general behavioral symptoms. It is noteworthy that this dog showed the weakest reaction concerning food intake behavior. Its food consumption even improved during the last two weeks of the main phase. This was a very important observation correlated to dog no. 6 and 8 that did not show relevant symptoms. From this, it can be said that simply because the animal shows no symptoms does not mean that the animal is doing well. It can be assumed that a lower food intake represents a reduced wellbeing of the animal, even though other symptoms are not present.

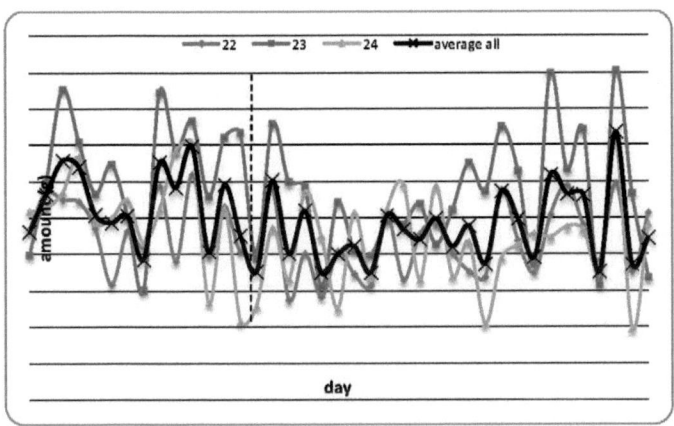

Chart 5.23: Average DFI of male group 2

Food intake of animal no. 23 (red) and no. 22 (blue) decreased slightly after the first day of the main phase and increased again after day 9 of the main phase. In this example, it was difficult to make a clear distinction between a normal and an abnormal feeding behavior, because both animals already had single days of low food intake in the pretest. The irregularity could be part of their normal feeding pattern.

In the case of male group 2, a change of the feeding pattern may be detected by analyzing other parameters of the feeding behavior, e.g. VpD or MDT.
For example, an increased number of VpD could be observed in animals that showed a reaction towards the test substance or environmental circumstances. Dogs that eat less in one visit may visit the feeder more often in order to eat the same amount of food. Thus, their changed feeding pattern would not show up in the amount of food intake but in the number of VpD.
Furthermore, the MDT may increase. Animals need more time to eat the same amount of food in the main phase than the pretest, if they were affected.

Male dogs of group 2 of study D had a steady number of VpD as well as a steady MDT. It was assumed that, because no food parameters had changed, the dogs were fine.

In analog to the results of no impact on food intake, there were also no symptoms documented in male group 2. Table 5.6 contains the documented symptoms of two dogs of this group.

Table 5.6: Symptoms of two animals of the male group 2

Animal no.	Sign Type	Sign	Modifier	Firstday	Lastday	Duration (days)
22	NORMAL	No remarkable clinical observations		1	27	27
	EYES	Discharge	Directional:both	28	30	3
23	NORMAL	No remarkable clinical observations		1	20	20
	EYES	Dried material around	Directional:both	21	22	2
	EYES	Discharge	Directional:both	23	23	1
	EYES	Dried material around	Directional:both	24	30	7

The symptom *dried material around the eyes* was valued as having no impact on the food intake.

Unlike in group 2, the higher concentration of the test substance in group 3 as well as group 4 of both sexes had a clear and significant impact on food intake (p <0.025). Due to the similar feeding patterns of group 3 and 4, only group 4 is demonstrated in the next chart. Group 1 of both sexes is added in chart 5.24 to highlight the impact of the test substance on the feeding pattern.

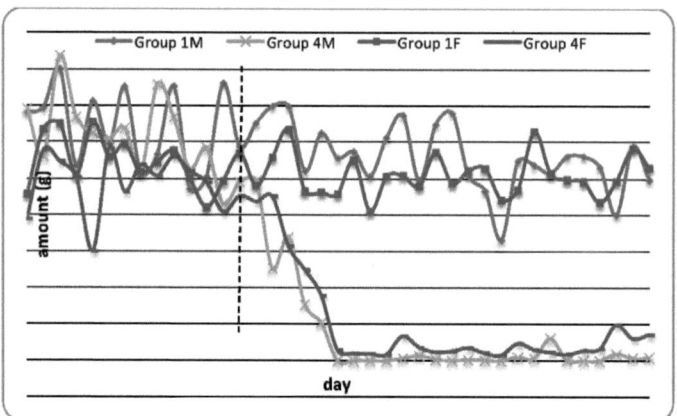

Chart 5.24: Average daily food intake compared between group 1 and 4 of both sexes

This chart gives an overview of groups 1 and 4 of males and females' food intake. The lines for the control group 1 of both sexes (blue male, red female) look very similar.
Food intake of group 4 (violet) of both sexes slightly decreased during the first week, but a clear impact was not seen before day 5, when food intake rapidly decreased to almost zero grams.

Dogs with no food intake after the first week were fed manually with wet food. These data were not included in the analysis, because the manual feeding was an artificial intervention. The dogs would not have eaten if no wet food had been offered. Besides, only the DFI was available. MDT and VpD could not be recorded by manually feeding

Other symptoms would be expected where such a strong impact on food intake induced by the test substance appeared. The symptoms of two animals based on the male group 4 are documented in table 5.11 and 5.12 and stand for the whole group 4 of both sexes.

Table 5.7: Symptoms of one male dog of high dose group 4

Animal no.	Sign Type	Sign	Modifier	Firstday	Lastday	Duration (days)
29	NORMAL	No remarkable clinical observations		1	13	13
	NEUROMUSCULAR	Motor activity decreased	Grade: slight	11	11	1
	NOSE	Discharge	Color: green	12	13	2
	SKIN/FUR	Swelling	Location: Snout/lip	13	30	18
	EYES	Discharge	Directional: both	14	14	1
	EYES	Eyelid(s) partially closed	Directional: both	14	19	6
	EYES	Dried material around	Directional: both	18	18	1
	SKIN/FUR	Discolored	Color: white, Location: head	18	30	13
	EYES	Eyelid(s) partially closed	Directional: both	21	30	10
	FECES/URINE	Feces mucoid		22	23	2
	FECES/URINE	Feces with apparent blood		22	23	2
	SKIN/FUR	Reddened	Location: Snout/lip	25	30	6
	NEUROMUSCULAR	Recumbency		26	26	1
	NEUROMUSCULAR	Motor activity decreased	Grade: slight	26	30	5
	LIMBS	Limping	Limb: forelimb, left	26	30	5

Surprisingly, even with such a clear impact on the food intake, practically no relevant symptoms were observed.
On day 11 and on day 26 to 30 neuromuscular symptoms were seen in dog 29. The amount eaten had already slowly decreased from day 0 and reached zero grams on day 7 for this particular dog. Four days later the symptoms appeared. The other symptoms listed in table 5.7 and 5.8 were not relevant with respect to the feeding behavior.

Table 5.8: Symptoms of a male dog of high dose 4

Animal no.	Sign Type	Sign	Modifier	Firstday	Lastday	Duration (days)
32	NORMAL	No remarkable clinical observations		1	1	1
	EYES	Discharge	Directional: right	1	3	3
	GENERAL BEHAVIOR	Licking excessively		2	2	1
	NORMAL	No remarkable clinical observations		4	16	13
	EYES	Dried material around	Directional: both	17	30	14
	SKIN/FUR	Discolored	Color: white, Location: head	18	30	13
	EYES	Eyelid(s) partially closed	Directional: both	19	19	1
	APPEARANCE	Thin appearance		20	24	5
	SKIN/FUR	Reddened	Location: Snout/lip	22	30	9
	SKIN/FUR	Swelling	Location: Snout/lip	22	30	9

In dog no.32 it seemed even more obvious that symptoms and deviations from the normal food intake did not correlate with one another.
This dog did not show any symptoms that could have indicated decreased food consumption.

In female group 4, there were also neurological symptoms documented on single days. In one female, vomiting was documented on day 6, 14, 16, and 17. Vomiting was also noticed in female group 1. It was not possible to say, whether vomiting had an influence on food intake due to its occurrence in control and test-item treated groups.

Timeslots

A similar situation with the shifts of the timeslots, which was previously described in study B was also observed in this study example D.
In study B, the dogs skipped their morning meals during the first week of the main phase.
In this study, the dogs of group 4 and group 3 of both sexes started to skip their morning meals after the first week. They still exhibited some food intake in the afternoon or evening. With further treatment with the test substance, afternoon and evening meals were skipped as

well as the study progressed. In contrary to other studies, e.g. study C, the test substance appeared to have a delayed effect on the food intake. In this case, a correlation of the skipped single meals due to the drug-induced effect was easier to make. The drug-induced effect was stronger and affected all test substance treated groups.

Duration of effect in the recovery

In most studies where an impact on the feeding patterns was observed, food intake of group 4 went back to baseline or at least increased to an acceptable amount in the recovery phase. However, in study D, the animals recovered only slowly from the main phase and DFI remained low. This is shown in an overview in chart 5.25.

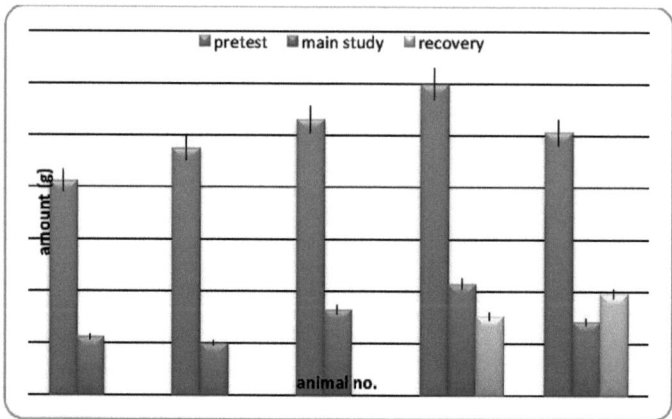

Chart 5.25: Average of DFI of female group 4 in pretest, main phase and recovery; (error bars with 5%)

Chart 5.25 illustrates the average of DFI in the three different study phases; pretest, main phase and recovery phase. The DFI of the pretest (blue) was clearly higher than in the other two phases. It was noted that the food intake in the recovery (green) was not higher than in the main phase (red). This may have been due to the previous treatment with the test substance.

5.2.5 Fifth example: Study E with an increasing food consumption

Based on the results of the sixteen studies, it can be said that most dogs slightly increased their food intake from week to week within the whole study. A slow increase in food intake occurred more frequently in control groups than in other test-item treated groups. Normally, at the end of the main phase, the amount of food was up to 100g higher than at the beginning of the pretest. This non-significant observation was made in groups that did not show a drug-induced impact on food intake.

In this last example, however, a clear and significant ($p<0.015$) increase in food intake could be observed soon after the beginning of the main phase. There was a dosage-proportional increase in food intake, most visibly in the highest dose group, i.e. in group 4 (p-value < 0.018).This implies that the impact was most likely drug-induced.
The effect was more prominent in females. Male dogs already ate their maximum of 450g during the pretest and continued with the same daily amount in the main phase. The mean values of the male dogs in the pretest and the main phase were almost the same, but might have increased if the animals had been given *ad libitum* access to food.

From day 0 onwards, food intake of female group 4 increased every day for the first two weeks before it slowly decreased at the end of the main phase. It is possible that the dogs adapted to the test substance's effect, resulting in a reduced food intake at the end of the main phase.
The food intake of the other groups increased too, but not as quickly and distinctly as seen in female group 4. This effect is illustrated in charts 5.26 and 5.27.

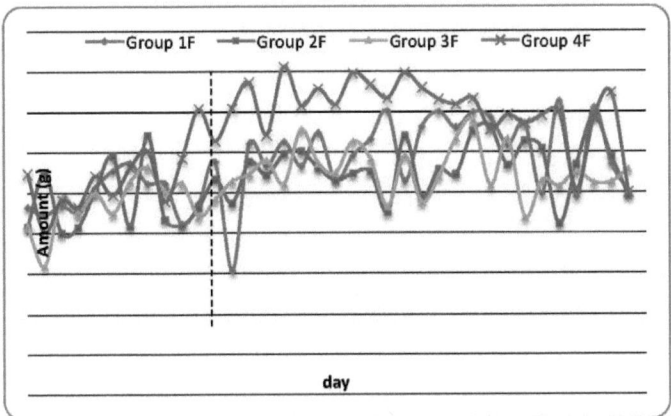

Chart 5.26: Average DFI of female group 1-4 of the example study

In chart 5.26, food intake of all four female groups increased in the main phase. Group 4 (violet) though, increased up to 400g per day, while the other female groups stayed of a lower level of daily food intake. The marked increase of food intake in the main phase is also illustrated in the bar chart 5.27.

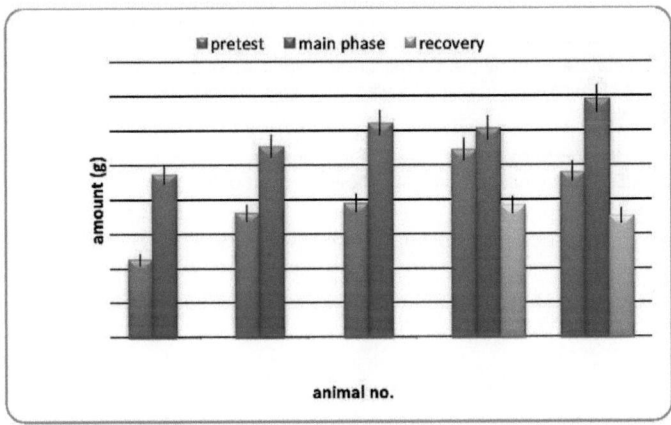

Chart 5.27: Mean values of DFI of all five animals (1-5) of female group 4, divided into pretest, main phase and recovery; (error bars with 5%)

The blue bars represent the mean values of the DFI of the animals in the pretest of female group 4. The red bars are the mean values of the DFI in the main phase and the green bars the mean values of the DFI in the recovery phase. As mentioned earlier, only two animals entered the recovery phase. This is why females number 1 to 3 have no green bar.

The DFI of the main phase were clearly higher than the DFI of the pretest and the recovery. Only female no. 4 had no clear increase. In the recovery phase (green) food intake of animal no. 4 and 5 was even lower than in the pretest. The low food intake in the recovery could also be observed in male group 4 in chart 5.28.

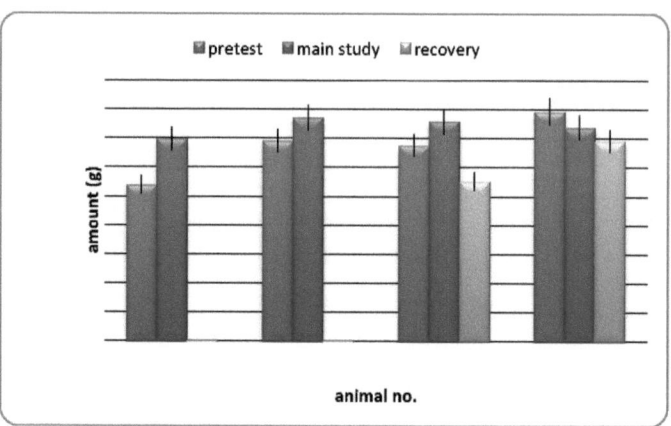

Chart 5.28: Average total food intake of all four male dogs (1-4) of group 4, divided into pretest, main phase and recovery; (errors bars with 5%)

As mentioned previously, the effect in males was not so obvious and probably due to the limited food allowance of 450g per day. In chart 5.28 another interesting observation was made.
Males had a slightly higher average of food intake in the main phase compared to the pretest. In the recovery, however, when test substance was no longer administered, food intake decreased which can be seen by the shorter green bars in chart 5.28. The test substance-related effect of increasing food intake was no longer present and the dogs went back to a lower food intake.

Even more evident than the increase in food intake of the females of group 4, as seen earlier in chart 5.27, was the MDT of the male group 4, as shown in chart 5.29.

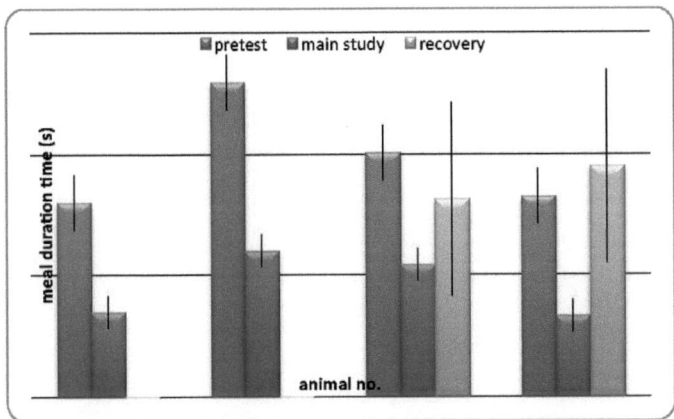

Chart 5.29: Mean values of MDT of male group 4 (1-4), divided into pretest, main phase and recovery; (error bars with 5%)

When comparing the average of the MDT of the pretest with the main phase the dogs ate visibly faster during the main phase.
The average of MDT of the recovery phase was also worthy of mention. In chart 5.28, it was noted that the food intake of male group 4 in the recovery phase was smaller than in the main phase. Instead of an expected shorter MDT due to the smaller amount of food, the MDT increased in the recovery.

The female dogs clearly ate more in the main phase and the male dogs ate significantly faster ($p < 0.04$) in the main phase compared to the pretest and the recovery. This effect was most likely drug-induced.

This conclusion was supported by a comparison of food intake and MDT of male group 4 with male group 1, starting with the food intake of group 1. Group 1 did not show a deviation of the feeding behavior between the three different study phases. The following chart shows the food intake of group 1.

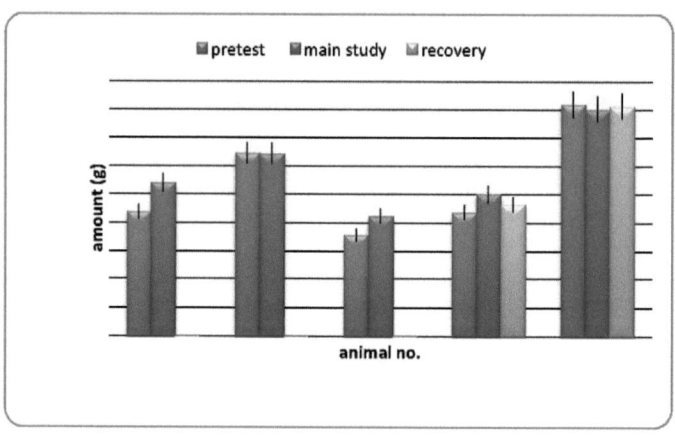

Chart 5.30: Mean values of DFI of male group 1 (1-5), divided into pretest, main phase and recovery; (error bars with 5%)

All five dogs of male group 1 ate steadily during the whole study. The mean values of the pretest, the main phase and the recovery were more or less the same. Even though animal no. 1-4 could have eaten more, they remained steady in the pretest and the main phase.

Chart 5.31 that contains the MDT looks the same as chart 5.30.

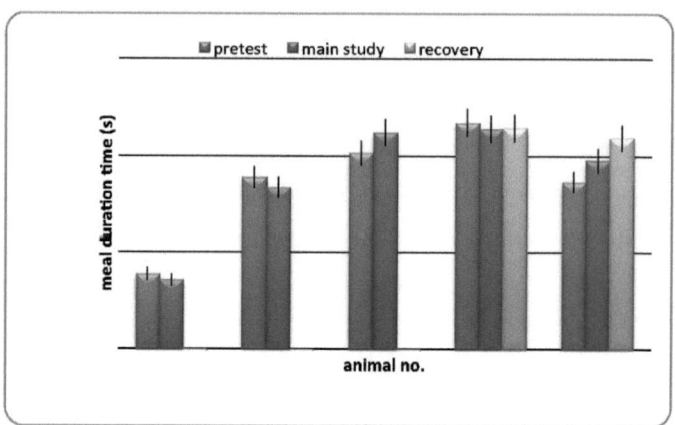

Chart 5.31: Mean values of MDT of male group 1 (1-5), divided into pretest, main phase and recovery (error bars with 5%)

The MDT of each individual animal during the main phase was as high as that seen for the same animal during the pretest for all five animals.

Eleven of the sixteen studies showed that a decrease in food intake was usually not accompanied by any symptoms. Low food intake and concurrent symptoms were less common. Thus, one can conclude that studies, which ascribe importance to symptoms, such as those that have been mentioned in these sixteen studies, miss the opportunity to include the relevance of changes in food intake behavior. It is particularly important to recognize a change in the feeding pattern as a symptom that may relate to the test substance. Deviations of the normal feeding behavior may be early signs of reduced wellbeing.

In this study, however, symptoms occurred in group 4 of both sexes; especially symptoms of the neuromuscular type. The neuromuscular signs to decrease food intake were not as strong as the drug-induced effect to increase food intake and hence did not influence the feeding patterns.

For each sex of group 4, one animal was chosen to illustrate the symptoms that appeared.

Table 5.9: symptoms of one male dog of high dose group 4

Animal no.	Sign Type	Sign	Modifier	First day	Last day	Duration (days)
179	NEUROMUSCULAR	Motor activity increased	Grade: marked	1	1	1
	NEUROMUSCULAR	Muscle tone reduced	Grade: slight	1	2	2
	NEUROMUSCULAR	Uncoordinated movement	Grade: marked	1	3	3
	NEUROMUSCULAR	Uncoordinated movement	Grade: slight	4	4	1
	NEUROMUSCULAR	Uncoordinated movement	Grade: marked	14	14	1
	NEUROMUSCULAR	Uncoordinated movement	Grade: slight	15	15	1
	NEUROMUSCULAR	Uncoordinated movement	Grade: slight	21	24	4
	NEUROMUSCULAR	Uncoordinated movement	Grade: slight	28	30	3
	NEUROMUSCULAR	Motor activity increased	Grade: marked	1	1	1
	NEUROMUSCULAR	Muscle tone reduced	Grade: slight	1	2	2
	NEUROMUSCULAR	Uncoordinated movement	Grade: marked	1	3	3
	ORAL / TEETH	Salivation		4	6	3
	ORAL / TEETH	Salivation		8	11	4
	EYES	Eyelid(s) partially closed	Directional: both	11	13	3
	NEUROMUSCULAR	Uncoordinated movement	Grade: marked	14	14	1
	NEUROMUSCULAR	Uncoordinated movement	Grade: slight	15	17	3
	NEUROMUSCULAR	Uncoordinated movement	Grade: marked	21	23	3
	ORAL / TEETH	Salivation		23	23	1
	NEUROMUSCULAR	Uncoordinated movement	Grade: slight	28	30	3

Table 5.10: Symptoms of one female dog of high dose group 4

Animal no.	Sign Type	Sign	Modifier	First day	Last day	Duration (days)
162	NORMAL	No remarkable clinical observations		1	2	2
	NEUROMUSCULAR	Uncoordinated movement	Grade: marked	1	3	3
	NEUROMUSCULAR	Muscle tone reduced	Grade: slight	2	2	1
	GENERAL BEHAVIOR	Trembling		3	9	7
	NEUROMUSCULAR	Motor activity decreased	Grade: slight	10	10	1
	NEUROMUSCULAR	Uncoordinated movement	Grade: marked	11	11	1
	NEUROMUSCULAR	Uncoordinated movement	Grade: slight	14	14	1
	NEUROMUSCULAR	Uncoordinated movement	Grade: marked	15	15	1
	NEUROMUSCULAR	Uncoordinated movement	Grade: slight	21	23	3
	NEUROMUSCULAR	Uncoordinated movement	Grade: marked	24	24	1
	NEUROMUSCULAR	Uncoordinated movement	Grade: slight	28	29	2

In table 5.9 the symptoms of a male dog and in table 5.10 the symptoms of a female dog of the high dose group (group 4) are presented.
The most common symptom was "uncoordinated movement" and the severity was scored as "slight" and "marked".
Other symptoms such as "motor activity increased/decreased" or "muscle tone reduced" were also recorded, but less often. Vomiting was only recorded in two animals of female group 4.
The symptoms appeared on the first day of the main phase and lasted throughout the whole phase.

Body weight

Females of group 4 showed an increase of more than 1kg of body weight; it rose from 7.8kg to 8.9kg most likely due to the increased food intake. The body weight of male group 4 increased as well, but only 500g on average.
The females lost between 500g and 1kg within the four weeks of the recovery due to the lower food intake. Thus, the animals more or less returned to their inital body weight they had at the beginning of the pretest.

Males of group 4 also had a lower food intake during the recovery, but none of them lost weight. One dog even gained weight despite eating less.

This indicates that body weight data without the information of the food intake does sometimes not give the right impression to the animals state of health.

5.4 Total visits

The number of VpD included only the visits where eating occurred and that were summarized as a meal. All dogs tended to visit the feeder without eating anything. These visits were defined as empty visits. Adding the empty visits and the ones with food intake results in the total visits per day. A deviation of the total visits was observed in studies with an impact on food intake.

Dogs entered the feeder between 1 to over 200 times a day, but not all visits were combined with food intake as you can see in figure 4.12. The visits with no food intake varied depending on the phase of the study and dog.
Some dogs reacted very clearly to the new study phases and the phase was identified by the change of number of total visits (including visits of no food intake and visits with food intake), which is visualized in the following two charts.

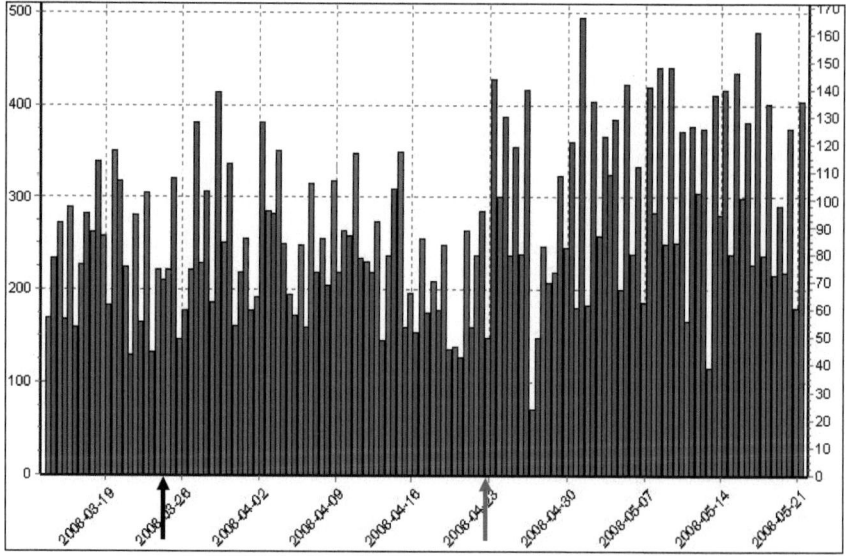

Chart 5.32: DFI and total visits of one dog for all three study phases; pretest, main phase and recovery: *Black arrow=start of the main phase; violet arrow=start of the recovery phase*

In chart 5.32, the amount of food is illustrated with red bars and the visits with green bars. The black arrow marks the start of the main phase and the blue arrow the start of the recovery. The start of the recovery was easily identified by the increased number of total visits resulting in higher green bars. There was also a short sequence of increased visits at the beginning of the main phase. The average of the total number of visits in the recovery was 127 times while in the main phase it was only 78 and in the pretest 71 times.

In the next chart, the opposite effect with lower visits is demonstrated.

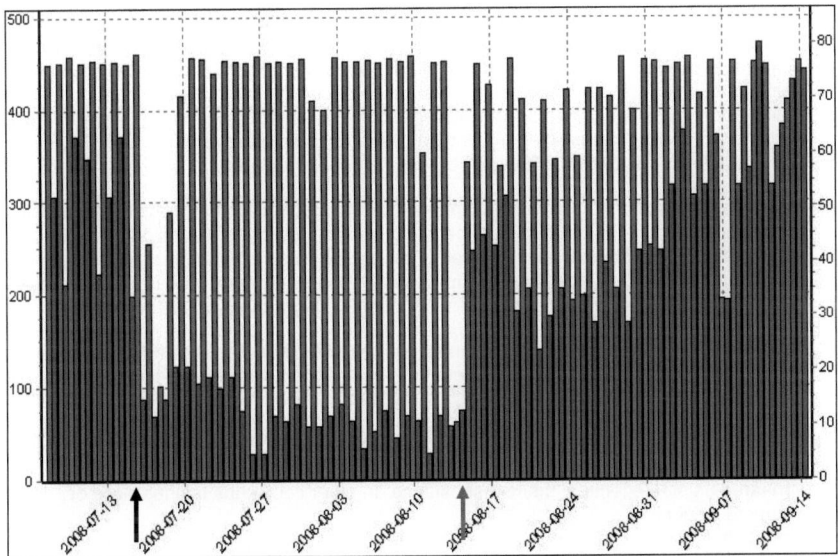

Chart 5.33: DFI and total visits of one dog for all three study phases; pretest, main phase and recovery: *Black arrow=start of the main phase; violet arrow=start of the recovery phase*

In this chart, it can be seen that the dog ate almost every day its 450g with some exceptions. The black arrow again marks the start of the main phase. From the first day on, the number of visits was clearly decreased. It seemed like the dog only entered the dog feeder to eat. The number of visits increased again in the recovery phase which is marked with the blue arrow. While the dog went into the dog feeder on average 52 times a day in the pretest, it only entered it 15 times a day in the main phase. In the recovery phase, it went up again to 45 visits a day. In this case, it can be assumed that the dog was affected by the treatment with the test substance, but no clear statement can be made due to the absence of statistical evidence.

The total visits data can be helpful if no software is available to allow an evaluation of the single meals. I did not analyze the total visits into more detail and no exact assessment on how often these situations appear could be made.

5.5. Symptoms

I included symptoms that appeared to have a possible influence on food intake. Some symptoms only appeared on one day, other symptoms were noted on several days in a row. Other symptoms that did not correlate with the test substance treatment e.g. bite wounds or scratches are not mentioned here.

An overview of all symptoms is given below with explanations of why these symptoms were chosen. The symptoms are categorized in main groups.

- **Gastrointestinal problems:** Gastrointestinal disorders are a daily problem in clinical practice and can be accompanied by nausea, reduced food intake or anorexia. Vomiting right after eating may induce CTA. Gastrointestinal symptoms are common in toxicology studies.
  Observed symptoms were salivation, vomiting, and diarrhea. In oncology studies, effects on food intake appeared progressively. Vomiting was noticed in fifteen studies and diarrhea in ten studies. Salivation was observed in all studies.

- **General behavior:** The general behavior of the dogs was observed daily. Behavioral changes such as disorientation, excessive licking or circling can distract the animals from eating and may cause lower food intake. An excessive exercise e.g. circling may even end in an increased required energy intake. Trembling and head shaking may disturb the animal while it eats. Symptoms were observed in eleven studies.

- **Neuromuscular:** Neuromuscular symptoms such as decreased/increased motor activity, recumbency, clonic-tonic convulsion, paddling movements, hyperextension of limbs, uncoordinated movements, and reduced or increased muscle tone may weaken the animal and lead to less exercise, less motion and may also hamper the dog while eating or it may induce nausea. In nine studies, neurological signs were observed.

- **Posture:** Abnormal posture of the animals, e.g. hunched position, distended abdomen, tilted head were also documented. Abnormal posture positions were observed in only three studies.

- **Limbs:** Injured or swollen legs and sore paws which are painful may decrease food intake due to reduced movement and pain. In certain studies, sore limbs or paws appeared as side effects of the test substance. In other cases, the injuries were of traumatic origin.
  Ten studies showed problems with legs or paws.

- **Respiration:** Similar to other symptoms respiration problems like panting or coughing could lead to reduced movement or discomfort, resulting in less food intake. In seven studies, symptoms related to the respiratory tract were documented.

The most common symptoms that were observed in all four dose groups throughout the sixteen studies were gastrointestinal problems, especially vomiting and salivation. Salivation appeared in all studies, especially within the first few days of administration. Salivation may be interpreted as a sign of nausea. Salivation was not only caused by the test substance, but also by the vehicle. This was evident as salivation was also observed in control group animals.

Due to the large number of the gastrointestinal observations, all three gastrointestinal symptoms are illustrated separately in the pie chart below. The other symptoms are not listed individually, but are summarized in their main groups.

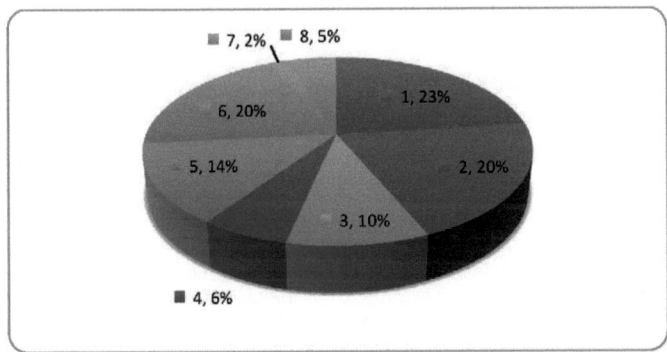

Chart 5.34: Appearance of the different symptoms in percentage: *1= salivation (23%), 2= vomiting (20%), 3= diarrhea (10%), 4= limbs (6%), 5= neurolog. signs (14%), 6= behavioral signs (20%),7= posture (2%), 8= respiration (5%); the percentage is referred to the total number of animals with or without symptoms*

222 (48.4%) out of 459 animals showed clinical symptoms of different types and severity grades.
As noted earlier in study E, some symptoms do not have to have an impact on food intake. In fact, in most of the sixteen studies, two possible situations were observed.
The first possibility was a reduced food intake at the beginning of the main phase with no observed symptoms. A few days later, when food intake started to increase, symptoms appeared. Food intake did not decrease again, when symptoms appeared (e.g. example 3, study C).
The other possibility was that the appearance of symptoms was observed within the first few days of the main phase, while food intake was more or less normal. After the symptoms disappeared, food intake either started to decrease or remained steady.
We rarely found a direct correlation between symptoms and the deviation on the feeding patterns. This observation was even reinforced by the statistical evaluation. Only one study showed a significant influence of symptoms on the daily food intake. A correlation between symptoms and the feeding patterns was rarely found.
This observation shows once more that food intake is an important parameter to establish the animal's wellbeing. Symptoms did not show up in all studies. If food consumption and, in particular, the feeding patterns are not considered, incorrect conclusions regarding the animal's wellbeing can be drawn.

6. Discussion

Animal studies are still essential in scientific research, medicines and development, and safety testing. Nevertheless, new alternative methods such as the study of cells and tissue grown in laboratories, computer modeled systems, and human patients, volunteers or populations decrease the number of animals used in experiments.

The statistical table of 2009 from the Swiss Federal Veterinary Office clarifies the numbers of animals used for testing in the different categories, namely industry, hospitals, fundamental research and others such as eco-toxicology, and non-medical research.
A decrease of animal testing can be observed in almost all categories. Only the eco-toxicology section had an increase from 2008 to 2009. Of all the animals used for animal testing 79% were rodents. Almost half of all animals were used in industry, which can be seen in table 6.1 and 6.2. In general, the total number of animals used for animal testing decreased from 2008 to 2009.

Table 6.1: Number of animals used in experiments 2009 (Swiss federal veterinary office)

Species	University, ETH, Hospitals	Federal, Cantons	Industry	Others	Total
Rodents	215170	3620	297382	29945	546117
Dogs	3112	241	1987	59	5399
Non-mammals	28074	25026	17817	47242	118159
Total	246356	28887	317186	77246	669675

Table 6.2: Number of animals used in experiments 2008 (Swiss federal veterinary office)

Species	University, ETH, Hospitals	Federal, Cantons	Industry	Others	Total
Rodents	220615	2772	315952	15682	555021
Dogs	2046	16	2491	70	4623
Non-mammals	40316	35817	13193	49383	138709
Total	262977	38605	331636	65135	698353

It can be seen that the number of dogs used for animal testing slightly increased from 2008 to 2009. The number of dogs used for industrial testing decreased from 2491 in 2008 to 1987 in 2009. More than 50% of the dogs for industrial purpose were used for pharmaceutical toxicology.

6.1 Thoughts regarding group housing dogs

In this study, the normal feeding behavior of group housed laboratory dogs was evaluated in a first step. The food intake data of the pretest phase served as the baseline to determine the normal feeding patterns. The feeding behavior was investigated by analyzing various parameters, such as the daily food intake (DFI), the meal duration time (MDT), the visits per day (VpD) or the timeslots of the meals. In a next step, the feeding patterns of the pretest phase were compared with the ones of the main phase and the recovery phase to document and interpret any deviations from the normal feeding patterns.
It was the aim of this study to show that the feeding patterns, defined by the various parameters, are helpful to detect deviations from the normal feeding behavior and thus deviations of the animals' state of health. This study shows that the feeding pattern is an important tool to estimate the animal's wellbeing. In most cases of studies with side effects,

an abnormal feeding behavior was the only clinical sign of a reduced wellbeing of the animals.

In the last couple of decades, it has been a target to enrich the animals' husbandry. One important step was the change from single housed to group housed husbandry.
Several studies were performed to investigate the differences of general behavior between single housed and group housed animals. It could be shown that group housed dogs developed less stereotypic behavior, e.g. circling (HETTS et al 1992), spent more time sniffing about the pen due to new scents, slept more and spent more time running around (HUBRECHT et al 1993).
It was also observed that group housed animals were more active with the presence of people (CAMPBELL et al 1988).

Since laboratory dogs in Switzerland were no longer single housed, it became more complicated to record individual food intake of dogs. HUBRECHT et al (1992) recommended not to separate the dogs for feeding. Instead, the value of food consumption data should be considered.

It has to be said that food consumption is an essential parameter in toxicology studies. The dose range finding studies just give one example, why food consumption should be documented.
As mentioned in section 3.4, toxicological tests are necessary for the drug's safety and to evaluate target organ toxicity. At the beginning of a dose range finding study, it is not known what kind of and when symptoms may appear. A deviation of the feeding behavior may be one of the first parameters that can be observed, if the dose range level approaches the toxicological dose.

To record individual food consumption, group housed dogs have to be either separated while feeding or only food consumption of a whole group is recorded. The documentation of food consumption of a group is less accurate and does not reflect the animal's individual feeding behavior. In addition, if the animals are fed manually, only the daily food intake is recorded and no exact evaluation of the daily feeding behavior is possible.

As shown by several examples throughout this study, the other parameters, e.g. the MDT revealed or even highlighted a drug-induced impact on food intake. Study E in the results section is the best example to illustrate this. Food consumption increased clearly in females, but only slightly in males, as explained in the example. Now, looking at the MDT of male group 4, it was clearly shorter in the main phase compared to the pretest and the recovery phase. Due to the daily limit of 450g, the food intake of male group 4 could not clearly increase. Without the MDT, the impact of the test substance on the feeding behavior of male group 4 would not have been in evidence.

The feeding behavior is also helpful to investigate the strongest effect of Cmax of a test substance on the animals. Dogs that are used to free access to food usually split their meals in three to four single meals. The majority of the dogs had at least one meal in the morning. It was observed that most animals had a decreased food intake in the morning within the first few days of the main phase. This could have been either drug-induced or stress-induced. These dogs tended to eat more frequently later on during the day.
It is known that dogs that are fed once daily get used to the situation and eat the whole amount at one time. Nevertheless, it does not reflect the dogs' natural feeding behavior.
For example, in Novartis Pharma Basel, before the dog feeders were implemented and when the dogs were fed manually, they only had three hours time to eat.
If the dogs were fed in the morning, they may not have eaten at that time due to the drug-induced effect. They could not eat later on, because food was removed after three hours. This means that the data for food intake of animals that are fed manually may be less accurate.

In addition, as seen in example D, a test substance can have a delayed impact. The dogs in study D started to skip their morning meals after the first few days, but still had food intake in the afternoon and evening. This could not be observed in manually fed animals, if feeding time is restricted to a certain time.

The problem of documenting food consumption in group housed dogs was solved at Novartis Pharma Basel by automated feeding machines as already explained in section 2. This way, dogs did not have to be separated while individual ongoing recording of food consumption was still possible. With the automated feeding system, the dogs could live out their natural feeding behavior. The recording of the MDT and the VpD as well as the single meals and the single meal duration time for each day and each animal is recorded with this system. Other parameters, such as the feeding rate (amount/time) are recorded as well. In my study, I did not use the feeding rate due to the high number of incorrect data caused by animals sleeping in the feeder.

Nevertheless, some disturbing factors that may occur in group housed animals and may have an influence on their feeding behavior should be considered when evaluating the data:

- Group behavior and dominance: depending on the group composition, hierarchic encounters could be observed and lower ranking animals were suppressed by dominant dogs in females and males. Some low ranking dogs did not dare to enter the feeder or were chased away.
- Some dogs tended to eat very variable amounts with a range of between 100 to 200g from day to day. This behavior was observed in control groups as well as in test item-treated groups and dogs that currently were not used for a study. It was not possible to say, if this feeding behavior may have occurred as well in single housed dogs.
- Distraction by other dogs e.g. when they were playing around. That could increase the VpD, or decrease the amount eaten during the day.
- Size of the group: Differences between small (two animals) and larger groups (five animals) could be observed. Smaller groups seemed to be more variable in food intake than larger groups. This was not statistically proved and is my subjective opinion.
- Any regrouping or reduction of the dogs could influence their feeding behavior
- The presence of people distracted the animals from eating
- Observations from animal keepers inside Novartis showed that some long-term animals behaved with a more aggressive attitude towards their conspecifics when a new animal keeper started to work in the animal husbandry part. The behavior lasted for one to two months, before the routine settled back down. Deviations of the feeding behavior during this time may be expected. No data was available to prove this observation.

6.2 Observations of daily food intake in the pretest, main phase, and the recovery phase

The data of sixteen regulatory studies was analyzed. As mentioned earlier in section 4, the studies had to fulfill certain criteria for this analysis. The most important criteria were the length of the study and the amount of dogs. Studies of less than two weeks did not deliver enough information. The groups had to contain at least three dogs of each sex to be comparative. In my analysis, the control and the high dose groups contained five dogs of each sex with a few exceptions.

I first tried to separate the studies into groups by the indication/therapeutic area of the compound being tested, e.g. all oncology studies together. This way, I expected to see any similarities in the feeding behavior when comparing the results between studies of same indication. However, the presentation turned out to be inappropriate as there were no similarities within the studies.

Taking the oncology-compound studies that were represented the most; every study had its own feeding profile. For example, in one oncology study, a clear impact could be seen; in

another one, no impact was observed and in some oncology studies, only part of the dogs of the same group showed a reaction. It was also possible that all dogs within a group behaved differently.
Another problem was that most indications within the sixteen studies were only represented once and no comparative study was available.

In a next step, I tried to classify the groups by their time to show any reaction on food intake caused by the test substance or the change of the daily routine. This means _immediate_ reaction right at the beginning of the main phase, _delayed_ reaction after a few days of the main phase or _no_ reaction. In some studies, all dogs of one group reacted the same way. In other studies, all dogs of one group showed different reactions to the test substance and this classification also turned out to be inappropriate.

Finally, the studies were classified into three different types of feeding patterns, also dependent on their reaction, but easier to summarize.

- Clear impact: all animals of a group showed a reaction, including males and females
- Irregular impact: certain animals of the same group showed a reaction
- No impact: none of the animals showed a reaction caused by the test substance

To summarize the reactions of all dose groups, the most common was the "*irregular impact*" - situation, occurring in fifteen out of sixteen studies followed of the "*clear impact*" -situation", mainly high dose groups of both sexes. "*No impact*" was the situation that was observed the least. Noteworthy is that more control groups showed an "*irregular impact*"- than a "*no impact*" reaction.

These observations led to the conclusion that the majority of the dogs were disturbed from their normal feeding behavior by several factors, not only by the drug-induced impact.

Males and females were allocated in the same room on opposite sides. One may assume that females in heat could have had a possible effect on the food consumption of males. In addition, females in heat would have eaten less. No such correlation could be demonstrated in my study.

Another point that had to be clarified was the time of year, when the study was performed. RASHOTTE et al (1984) described a lower food intake in summer compared to colder days in their study. Their animals were outside the whole time.
In Novartis, the dogs also had access to outdoor areas at ambient temperatures. The studies were divided into spring, summer, autumn and winter. The mean values of the DFI of the dose groups in the same season time were compared with the other seasons. No seasonal influence was observed on the food consumption of dogs. One can assume that the dogs may have spent more time inside than outside which may explain why no influence of the season on the food intake was observed.
There may have been an influence on individual animals; however I did not analyze that level of detail.

6.2.1 Pretest
The pretest phase lasted in general for one week. At the beginning of this week, dogs were regrouped and allocated to new rooms. Several in-life examinations as described in 3.7 were performed during this week.
The pretest was meant to deliver the baseline for the comparison with the other phases, especially the main phase.
It has to be said that not all dogs delivered reliable results. Some dogs tended to eat very variably and interpretations of their feeding behavior were difficult or not possible.
One possibility for the variable feeding pattern could have been the in-life examinations and the new conditions due to regrouping and allocating to new rooms.

Another possibility to consider was the irregularity reflecting certain dogs' normal feeding behavior.
The variable food intake fluctuated from day to day, mostly within a range of 100g.
In addition, the irregular feeding behavior was not only observed during the pretest, but also during the main phase and the recovery and even in dogs that did not run in a study at that moment. Including all observations, I assumed that the irregular feeding pattern reflected the normal behavior in certain dogs, if it lasted throughout the three study phases. It was not triggered by stress or other influences. Due to my observations, I defined fluctuations of 100g from day to day were part of the normal feeding behavior in most dogs. In addition, the dogs had a limit of 450g, which corresponded to double the amount needed for their required energy intake. Probably on one day they ate more than their required energy intake demanded, resulting in a lower food intake the next day.
There were no other reasons found for the irregular feeding behavior. The variable food intake was more common in females, but males also had a variable food intake.
Dogs with an irregular feeding behavior in the pretest complicated the comparison of the feeding patterns between the different study phases.

Novelty is a strong stressor (Dantzer et al 1983) which as well influences feeding patterns. Plasma cortisol concentrations are a common factor to measure stress, especially long-term stress. This was also emphasized by a study of CLARK et al from 1997. In their study, the plasma cortisol values in dogs were high within the first week of the study, regardless of treatment condition. At the end of the first week, the plasma cortisol level then gradually decreased.

The effect of stress can be reduced, if the animal is conditioned gradually to handling procedures (HUTSON 1993), for example for ECG-recording. From my own observations, it could be said that most dogs that were not used to ECG-recordings reacted anxiously and a high heart rate was measured. It may be worth training the planned examinations with the animals before performing them in the study.

Considering these points, the beginning of the pretest can be stressful and distracting, which results in a fluctuating food intake and lasted in several animals up to one week.
In addition, in the guidelines of the workshop of LASA (**Guidance on the transport of laboratory animals 2004**), the authors recommend an adapting time of at least three days when the animals are moved to new allocations.
Generally, in most of the studies performed in Novartis Pharma Basel, the dogs were moved to new rooms at the start of the pretest and did not get three more days to adapt. It has to be considered that the pretest stands for the baseline data of the animals' feeding behavior to compare with other study phases. Results of the feeding behavior in the pretest of animals that were not adapted yet may lead to incorrect conclusions.
Thus, in my opinion, the pretest phase was too short and should be prolonged to two weeks.

6.2.2 Main phase
Several reactions were observed at the beginning of the main phase due to the new processes and/or the test substance. The most common reaction was an irregular feeding pattern with a lower food intake within the first few days of the main phase as mentioned earlier. The daily rhythm of the pretest ended abruptly on day 0. A new routine with daily administrations, in-life examinations, and more intensive interactions between animal keepers and the dogs followed and could explain the reduced food intake.

In some dogs, nevertheless, feeding behavior became regular from the first day of the main phase on, as shown in study B in chart 5.17.
This regular feeding pattern was observed in 22 dogs, more likely in males. Only six females became steady at the beginning or after the first week of the main phase. This behavior led to the assumption that some dogs can deal with stress better than other dogs.

353 of the dogs were irregular during the pretest and the main phase with different ranges of fluctuation, whereby the irregularity of the food intake was more pronounced in the main phase.
Nevertheless, it was still possible to allocate most of the reactions to either drug-induced or stress-induced effects.
If the whole group of a study showed an impact on food intake, the deviation of the feeding behavior was associated to the effect of the test substance. If only part of the dogs of one group showed a reaction, it had to be carefully considered what caused the reaction. It depended on the dog's feeding pattern in the pretest. If the dog was already very variable in the pretest, the irregularity of the feeding pattern in the main phase was more likely its normal feeding attitude or it was caused by environmental distractions. A more regular pretest or a smaller range of fluctuation in the pretest compared to the main phase were more indicative for a distraction, either by the test substance or by stress due to the performance of the study.
In addition, if the reaction lasted only for one or two days, it was more likely caused by environmental distraction or the variable food intake of the animal. Longer lasting reactions were more likely associated with the test substance.

The impact on food intake of a test substance could be seen most likely within the first week of the main phase. In most studies the dogs adapted to the effect of the test substance after one week and their food intake increased again.

6.2.3 Recovery

There were only two dogs left during the recovery phase. The lower number of dogs may have delivered less reliable statistical results.

In most cases when dogs ate irregularly in the main phase they remained irregular in the recovery phase as well.
The fact that most dogs became or stayed variable during the recovery, even though no in-life examinations were performed until the last week of the recovery cannot be clearly explained. A reaction to the smaller group composition could be one reason. The dogs may have been less active, slept more, and they were less jealous about food. On the other hand, they may also have been less distracted from eating which would result in an increased or steady food intake.

The reactions in the recovery phase were less pronounced than in the main phase. It was observed that the majority of the 114 dogs had one to two days of low food intake in the transition period from the main phase to the recovery. This was most likely a reaction to processes at the end of the main phase. Dogs that did not enter the recovery phase were euthanized and used for autopsy while the recovery animals were left behind. The dogs reacted sensitively to this process and the new group composition.

I could observe different reactions in the recovery phase. In studies with a clearly lower food intake in the main phase, the dogs started to eat more step by step in the recovery phase. A reverse behavior was observed in studies, where no clear impact on food consumption could be measured. These dogs' food intake decreased during the recovery phase. Only in one study, I could associate the reduced food intake in the recovery to the effect of the test substance.

I concluded that the required energy intake in the recovery phase was lower than in the main phase. This would explain, why dogs from studies with no or only slight impact on the feeding behavior ate less in the recovery compared to the main phase. On the other hand, dogs that showed a strong reaction on the feeding behavior in the main phase by a lower food intake had to compensate their energy deficit, resulting in an increased food intake in the recovery.

In addition, dogs that had a higher food limit than others in the main phase due to an increased required energy intake ate less in the recovery. This was another indication that dogs had lower energy maintenance in the recovery phase.

The body weight of the dogs was another parameter which highlights this conclusion. Body weight was compared between the main phase and the recovery.
Only differences of body weight of more than 200g between the first and the last value of the main phase were defined as loss of body weight. The dogs lost between 300g and 1.5kg, whereby stronger loss of body weight was only observed in animals of group 4.

Five male dogs of group 1 and seventeen dogs of group 4 lost body weight during the main phase. No male dog lost body weight in the recovery.
There were nine females of group 1 and thirteen females of group 4 that lost body weight in the main phase. Another six animals lost body weight in the recovery, whereby three of the six animals gained weight in the main phase as a result of treatment with the test item and went back to their baseline value in the recovery.

The male dogs of the different control groups that lost body weight in the main phase did not have an increased food intake in the recovery, but still regained body weight in this phase. This observation was described in the second example, Study B. This is only speculation; however, the loss of body weight in control animals could lead one to the assumption that the control animals had a higher energy intake requirement in the main phase compared to the recovery.

It would be expected that animals that ate less and lost body weight in the main phase would eat more in the recovery to compensate their negative energy intake. Indeed, all animals that lost body weight in the main phase, except for one female, regained body weight or did not lose further body weight in the recovery phase. There was not always an association between increased food intake and regained body weight. The absence of drug administration and in-life examinations was possibly enough to reduce the dogs' energy maintenance.

6.2.4 Single meals
It was not always known at the beginning of a study what kind of effect the test substance could induce. Thus there were test substances with an immediate reaction on the food intake within the first week of the main phase. Other test substances, especially oncology compund-studies had a delayed effect on the food intake. It depended on the mechanism and its target cell effect of the test substance.

I divided the single meals in four timeslots to see, if the Cmax of the test substance correlated with a lower food intake within a certain time interval during the day or if the impact of the test substance was not related to time intervals. Some test substances may only have had a strong short lasting effect in the morning, while the effect of other test substances may have lasted throughout the whole day. Not all dogs ate in the morning. Some preferred to eat in the afternoon and evening. The afternoon and evening meals varied too much in their size. Only dogs with a constant pattern of the single morning meals could be compared. Otherwise distinctions of the normal rhythm could not be seen. The meaningful pattern was illustrated in the second example in charts 5.13 and 5.14.
To make a clear statement about the effect on single meals, the mean values of the test substance's concentration in the dog's plasma (toxicokinetic parameters) should be analyzed and compared with the single meal patterns.
Further, it was observed that control animals also showed an impact on the morning meals. Their meals became smaller within the first two to four days of the main phase. If control and high dose dogs of one study reacted the same way, the distinction between drug-induced and stress-induced effects of shifting was difficult.

6.2.5 DFI and visits

In accordance with reports from previous studies and observations (GV-SOLAS), our results showed a range of VpD from three to five times.
It was only a small number of animals visiting the feeder less than two or more than eight times per day. Only one dog was observed eating fourteen times on one day.
Due to a high number of VpD in certain dogs, I considered the intermeal interval chosen too short and a prolonged intermeal interval of fifteen minutes may have been better.

Stress or a reduced wellbeing was not only expressed as a fluctuation of the daily food intake, but also as a decreased or increased number of VpD, which was explained in the first example in chart 5.10 and in the third example in chart 5.21.
As you can see in chart 5.10, the VpD were higher at the beginning of the pretest and decreased after a few days, when they adapted to the daily routine and when daily food intake became more regular.
After a period of decreased food intake, the number of visits exceeded that of the pretest, but for the same or even a smaller amount, which was explained in chart 5.21.

I concluded that a distraction from the normal feeding behavior could also be seen in a deviation of the VpD. In certain cases, only the VpD changed, while DFI remained constant, as seen in chart 5.10. The parameter "VpD" was helpful by allowing a more sensitive analysis of the dog's feeding behavior, when no deviation of the DFI could be found.

6.2.6 DFI and MDT

Control dogs as well as dogs of the test substance-treated groups that were not affected by the compound had an increase of food intake from week to week throughout the three study phases, as mentioned at the beginning of the fifth example in section 5. The MDT on the other hand became significantly shorter, more pronounced in males than females. Healthy dogs needed less time to eat the same amount of food compared to dogs with a reduced wellbeing. This could be seen in the fifth example. The test substance had a food increasing effect. The male dogs in this example ate clearly faster in the main phase compared to the other two study phases.
The negative impact of the test substance on MDT was shown in chart 5.22 in the third example. The dog had to spend more time to eat a smaller amount of food. I concluded that the MDT was another parameter to be used to ascertain a dog's state of health. Even though the MDT of most dogs decreased with the reduced DFI, a prolonged MDT with a reduced or constant DFI could also be observed in certain dogs. This was a sign of a reduced wellbeing.

6.2.7 DFI and symptoms

As explained earlier, symptoms in most cases did not correlate with the deviations of the DFI and each animal had its own reaction to stress or the drug-induced effect.

When I started to analyze the studies, I expected a clear decrease of food intake in studies where severe or numerous symptoms were documented. Furthermore, I expected studies with slight deviations of food consumption in combination with only slight or no symptoms. During the analysis, I realized that it was more likely to be the other way around. In studies, where the strongest impact on food intake was observed only a few or no other symptoms were documented. Eleven studies showed a drug-induced impact on feeding behavior in part of the animal groups or in all animals within a dose group. The symptoms in the eleven studies occurred either one week later than the impact appeared or they registered only on single days.
Normally, the first observation of the drug-induced effect in the main phase was a decreased or no food intake. In most cases, food consumption recovered, which could be seen by an increase of the DFI. While food intake increased, symptoms appeared, but did not influence the food consumption. This scenario can be observed in 5.2.3 in the third example.

In general, neurological symptoms tended to have only a small effect on food consumption. The best example to demonstrate the weak influence of neurological symptoms can be observed in 5.2.5 in the fifth example.

In three studies out of the sixteen, symptoms and a decrease of food intake appeared within the same time frame, most commonly in the first week of the main phase.

For a more precise conclusion of how symptoms are influencing food consumption, more specific parameters, e.g. hormones or neurotransmitters have to be included in the analysis. Nevertheless, as explained above, a deviation of food intake was in most cases the only parameter that demonstrated the animal's state of health and should therefore be included into the documentation of symptoms.

6.2.8 Feeding behavior and pathological findings

I tried to find a correlation between reduced food intake and pathological findings. A deviation of the feeding behavior could not be correlated with pathological findings; only speculations could be made.

In certain studies where an impact could be seen, no pathological findings were found. In other studies, the pathological findings were found in control and dose groups. Another observation was that the animals had pathological findings of the gastrointestinal system and other organs, but did not show an abnormal feeding behavior. Due to these different results, a correlation seemed too vague to draw any conclusions from it.

6.2.9 Correlation between food intake and clinical parameters

At the beginning of this study, I considered comparing the daily food intake with the clinical parameters of hematology and clinical biochemistry. Blood samples were only taken 4 times within 9 weeks. As the samples were only taken on certain days and not more regularly, the results did not represent the situation over the whole study phase. Thus, I did not include the clinical parameters into the evaluation.

6.3 Conclusion

Food intake was influenced by various factors. One important influence was as expected, the test substance. But other factors such as changes of the daily routine, new group compositions, a short pretest phase and individual reactions had to be included as well, when evaluating the feeding behavior.
Referring to the tables in section 5, where the values of all dogs are listed it can be said that the dogs with reduced health ate more slowly and less.

The DFI was the most sensitive and robust parameter in my study to evaluate the feeding behavior, but other parameters such as the VpD and the MDT were important too, especially in cases with unclear results, e.g. when DFI remained steady. Referring to the tables 5.1 and 5.2 in section 5, it can be said that the dogs tend to eat less, slower and split into more single meals, if their wellbeing is reduced.
The feeding behavior should be included in the daily documentation and treated as a clinical symptom. Animals mostly ate less before more severe symptoms appeared. A reduced food intake is a sign of a decreased wellbeing of the animal.
It should also be considered to not only evaluate the DFI but also other parameters such as MDT and VpD. This is not possible when dogs are fed manually once daily. A more regular access to food should be provided to enrich the animals housing facilities. When the animals are fed with the Dogfeeder system, a more precise observation of the feeding behavior is possible and delivers more reliable results.

The observations and conclusions made during the evaluation are summarized once again:

1. Dogs did not eat as regularly as expected, which made it more difficult to interpret the results
2. Dogs showed different reactions, beginning with no impact on the feeding behavior to very strong reactions such as no food intake at all
3. The daily amount of food was the most important parameter to measure the dogs' wellbeing, but other parameters such as VpD, MDT and daily meal rhythm were helpful as well, especially in situations with no clear effect on the food intake
4. Lower food intake seldom correlated with the appearance of symptoms
5. Disturbance factors always have to be considered. For example group behavior, individual behavior
6. Fluctuations of the DFI during one or two days were considered more likely to stress or the dog's natural feeding behavior than to a drug-induced effect; a daily fluctuation of 100g was common
7. Males and females may react differently. In such cases, the concentration of the test item in the dogs' plasma should be compared between the two sexes for further conclusions
8. Compounds for same therapeutic area did not cause the same reactions on the feeding behavior
9. Feeding behavior is important and should be included when assessing the dogs state of health

7. References

AUSTRALIAN GOVERNMENT
Guidelines to promote the wellbeing of animals used for scientific purposes (2008)
The assessment and alleviation of pain and distress in research animals
http://www.nhmrc.gov.au/_files_nhmrc/publications/attachments/ea18.pdf

BEERDA BONNE, SCHILDER MATTHIJS B.-H., BERNADINA WILBERT, VAN HOOFF JAN A.R.A.M., DE VRIES HANS W., MOL JAN A.
Chronic Stress in Dogs Subjected to Social and Spatial Restriction: II. Hormonal and Immunological Responses
Physiology & Behavior 1999, Vol. 6 (2), pp 243-254

BRADSHAW JOHN W.S.
Sensory and experimental factors in the design of foods for domestic dogs and cats
Proceeding of the Nutrition Society 1991, Vol. 50, pp. 99-106,

BRADSHAW JOHN W.S.
The Evolutionary Basis for the Feeding Behavior of Domestic Dogs (Canis familiaris) and Cats (Felis catus)
The Waltham International Science Symposia 2006, Journal of Nutrition, pp. 1927-1931

BRUININX E.M., VAN DER PEET-SCHWERING C.M., SCHRAMA J.W., VEREIJKEN P.F., VESSEUR P.C., EVERTS H., DEN HARTOG L.A., BEYNEN A.C.
Individually measured feed intake characteristics and growth performance of group-housed weanling pigs; effects of sex, initial body weight, and body weight distribution within groups
Journal of Animal Science 2001, Vol. 79, pp. 301-308

CAMMACK K.M., LEYMASTER K.A., JENKINS T.G., NIELSEN M.K.
Estimates of genetic parameters for feed intake, feeding behavior, and daily gain in composite ram lambs
Journal of Animal Science 2005, Vol. 83, pp. 777-785

CAMPBELL S.A., HUGHES H.C., GRIFFIN H.E., LANDI M.S., MALLON F.M.,
Some effects of limited exercise on purpose-bred Beagles
Am. J. Vet. Res. 1988, Vol. 49, pp. 1298-1301

CHAUDHRI OWAIS, SMALL CAROLINE, BLOOM STEVE
Gastrointestinal hormones regulating appetite
Philosophical Transactions of the Royal Society 2006, Vol. 361, pp. 1187-1209

CHAPMAN C.R., CASEY K.L., DUBNER R., FOLEY K.M., GRACELY R.H., READING A.E.
Pain measurement: an Overview
Journal of Pain 1985, Vol 22, pp. 1-31

CHENG CHRISTINE A., GEOGHEGAN JUSTIN G., LAWSON D. CURTIS, BERLANGIERI SAM. U., AKWARI ONYE, PAPPAS THEODORE N.
Central and peripheral effects of CCK receptor antagonists on satiety in dogs,
The American Physiology Society 1993, pp. 219-223

CLARK DERELL J., RAGER DAWN R., CALPIN JANET P.
Animal Well-Being: I. General Considerations
Laboratory Animal Science 1997, Vol. 74, pp. 564-570

CLARK DERRELL J., RAGER DAWN R., CROWELL-DAVIS SHARON, AND EVANS DONALD L.
Housing and Exercise of Dogs: Effects on Behavior, Immune Function, and Cortisol Concentration
Laboratory Animal Science 1997, Vol. 47 (5), pp 500-510

DANTZER R., MORMEDE P.
Stress in farm animals: A need for reevaluation
Journal of American Science 1983, Vol. 57 (6), pp. 6-18

DEMARIA-PESCE VICTOR H., NICOLAIDIS STYLIÏANOS
Mathematical Determination of Feeding Patterns and its Consequences on Correlational studies,
Physiology & Behavior 1998, Vol. 65 (1), pp. 157-170

DRUG DISCOVERY
http://www.innovation.org/drug_discovery/objects/pdf/RD_Brochure.pdf

EUROPEAN AGENCY FOR THE EVALUATION OF MEDICINAL PRODUCTS (emeA)
Non-clinical safety studies for the conduct of human clinical trials for pharmaceuticals
ICH step 5 (CPMP/ICH/286/95, modification) 2000

EUROPEAN MEDICINES AGENCY
Non-Clinical safety studies for the conduct of human clinical trials and marketing authorization for pharmaceuticals: Note for guidance on non clinical safety studies for the conduct of human clinical trials and marketing authorization for pharmaceuticals (CPMP/ICH/286/95) 2009, http://www.emea.europa.eu

EWE K., KARBACH U.
Funktionen des Magen-Darm-Kanals
In: Physiologie des Menschen, Editor Schmidt Robert F. and Thews Gerhard, Springer-Verlag, 24. Auflage 1990, pp. 734-735

FEDERATION OF EUROPEAN LABORATORY ANIAML SCIENCE ASSOCIATIONS (FELASA) WORKING GROUP ON ANIMAL HEALTH
FELASA recommendations for the health monitoring of breeding colonies and experimental units of cats, dogs and pigs,
Report of the FELASA Working Group on Animal Health, Laboratory Animals 1998, Vol. 32, pp. 1-17

FLECKNELL P.A.
Refinement of animal use-assessment and alleviation of pain and distress
Laboratory animals 1994, Vol. 28, pp. 222-231

FREGLY M.J. 1980
On the spontaneous intake of NaCl solution by dogs
In: Biological and behavioral aspects of salt intake, Editor Kare M.R.,Fregly M.J., Bernard R.A, Academic Press New York 1980, pp. 55-68

GALOSY R.A., CLARKE L.K., MITCHELL J.H.
Cardiac changes during behavioral stress in dogs
American Journal of Physiology - Heart and Circulatory Physiology 1979, Volume 5 (5), pp. H750-H758

GEOGHEGAN JUSTIN G., CHENG CHRISTINE A., LAWSON CURTIS, NAPPAS THEODORE N.
The Effect of caloric load and nutrient composition on induction of small intestinal satiety in dogs
Physiology&Behavior 1997, Vol. 62 (1), pp. 39-42

GOETSCHEL ANTOINE F.
Kommentar zum Eidgenössischen Tierschutzgesetz; Verlag Paul Haupt Bern und Stuttgart 1986, pp. 16, 35-38

GESELLSCHAFT FÜR VERSUCHSTIERKUNDE (GV-SOLAS)
Ausschuss für Ernährung der Versuchstiere: Fütterungskonzepte und – Methoden in der Versuchstierhaltung und im Tierversuch 2009, p. 3

HART BENJAMIN L.
Biological basis of the behavior of sick animals
Neuroscience&Biobehavioral Reviews 1988, Vol. 12 (2), pp. 123-137

HART BENJAMIN L.
Breed and gender differences in behaviour
In: "domestic dog: its evolution, behaviour and interactions with people", Editor Serpell J., Cambridge University Press 1995, pp. 65-77

HETTS SUZANNE, CLARK DARELL J., CALPIN JANET P., ARNOLD CHERYL E., MATEO JILL M.
Influence of housing conditions on beagle behaviour
Applied Animal Behaviour Science 1992, Vol. 34, pp. 137-155

HOUPT KATHERINE A., SMITH SHARON L.
Taste Preferences and their Relation to Obesity in Dogs and Cats,
Canadian Veterinary Journal 1981, Vol. 22 (4), pp 77-81

HUBRECHT ROBERT C., SERPELL JAMES A., POOLE TREVOR B.
Correlates of pen size and housing conditions on the behavior of kenneled dogs
Applied Animal Behaviour Science 1992, Vol. 34, pp. 365-383

HULSEY MARTIN G., MARTIN ROY J.
A System for Automated Recording and Analysis of Feeding Behavior,
Physiology&Behavior 1991, Vol. 50, pp. 403-408

HUTSON G. D.
Behavioral principles of sheep handling
In: Assessment of stress during handling and transport, Editor T. Grandin, Journal of American Science 1997, Vol. 75, pp. 249-257

HYUN Y., ELLIS M., JOHNSON R.W.
Effects of feeder type, space allowance and mixing on the growth performance and feed intake pattern of growing pigs,
Journal of Animal Science 1998, Vol. 76, pp. 2771-2778

HYUN Y., ELLIS M., MCKEITH F.K., WILSON E.R.
Feed intake pattern of group-housed growing-finishing pigs monitored using a computerized feed intake recording system,
Journal of Animal Science 1997 Vol. 75, pp. 1443-1451

JANOWITZ HENRY D., GROSSMAN M.I.
Some factors affecting the food intake of normal dogs and dogs with esophagostomy and gastric fistula
Department of Clinical Science, University of Illinois 1949

JAENIG W.
Vegetatives Nervensystem
In: Physiologie des Menschen, Editor Schmidt Robert F. and Thews Gerhard, Springer-Verlag 1990, 24. Auflage, pp. 376-383

KIENZLE ELLEN, RAINBIRD ANNA
Maintenance Energy Requirement of Dogs: what is the Correct Value for the Calculation of Metabolic Body Weight in Dogs?
Journal of Nutrition 1991, Vol. 121, pp. 39-40

KITCHELL BARBARA E.
Anorexia and Polyphagia
In: Textbook of Veterinary Internal Medicine Vol. 1, Editor Ettinger Stephen J., W.B.Saunders Company 1989, pp. 15-17

KITCHELL R.L.
Dogs know what they like
Friskies Res. Dig. 1972, Vol. 8 (3), pp. 1-4

LABORATORY ANIMAL SCIENCE ASSOCIATION (LASA)
Guidance on dose level selection for regulatory general toxicology studies for pharmaceuticals
In collaboration with the National Centre for the Replacement, Refinement and Reduction of Animals in Research, 2009

LABORATORY ANIMAL SCIENCE ASSOCIATION (LASA)
Guidelines for the Transport of Laboratory Animals 2005, Vol. 39, pp. 1-39

LANGHANS WOLFGANG, SCHARRER E.
Regulation der Nahrungsaufnahme
In: Physiologie der Haustiere, Editor v. Engelhardt W., Enke Verlag Stuttgart 2000, pp. 409-421

LANGHANS WOLFGANG
Signals generating anorexia during acute illness
From: Symposium on "Eating", illness and the gut: is there a disorder in the house?"
Nutrition Society 2007, Vol. 66, pp. 321-330

LANGHANS WOLFGANG
Anorexia during Disease,
In: Neurobiology of food and fluid intake, 2nd edition, Vol. 14 of handbook of behavioral neurobiology, Kluwek Academics 2004

LEVINE ALLEN S., SIEVERT CHESTER E., MORLEY JOHN E., GOSNELL BLAKE A., SILVIS STEPHEN E.
Peptidergic regulation of feeding in the dog (Canis familiaris).
Peptides 1984, Vol 5 (4), 675-676,

LUTZ THOMAS, GEARY N.
The gut-brain axis in the control of eating. Appetite and Body Weight: Inegrative systems and the development of anti-obesity drugs,
Editor Cooper S.J., Kirkham T.C., associated Press, Elsevier 2006, pp. 143-166

MADRID JUAN A. MATAS PURA, SÁNCHEZ-VÁZQUEZ F. JAVIER, CUENCA EUGENIO
A Contact Eatometer for Automated Continuous Recording of Feeding Behavior in Rats
Physiology&Behavior 1995, Vol. 57 (1), pp. 129-134

MUSSA P.P., PROLA L.
Dog Nutrient Requirements: New Knowledge
Veterinary Research Communications 2005, Vol. 29, pp. 35-38

NATIONAL RESEARCH COUNCIL (US) COMMITTEE ON RECOGNITION OF PAIN IN LABORATORY ANIMALS
1 Pain in Research: General Principles and Considerations
In: Recognition and Alleviation of Pain in Laboratory animals, National Academies Press (US) 2009, Washington (DC), pp. 1-10
www.ncbi.nlm.nih.gov/books/NBK32655

NATIONAL RESEARCH COUNCIL (US) COMMITTEE ON RECOGNITION OF DISTRESS IN LABORATORY ANIMALS
2 Stress and Distress: Definitions
In: Recognition and Alleviation of Distress in Laboratory Animals, National Academies Press (US) 2008, Washington (DC), pp. 1-8
www.ncbi.nlm.nih.gov/books/NBK4027

NATIONAL RESEARCH COUNCIL (US) COMMITTEE ON RECOGNITION OF DISTRESS IN LABORATORY ANIMALS
3 Recognition and Assessment of Stress and Distress
In: Rooognition and Alleviation of Distress in Laboratory Animals, National Academies Press (US) 2008, Washington (DC), pp. 1-23
www.ncbi.nlm.nih.gov/books/NBK4033

NOVARTIS PHARMA AG
Research and development: drug discovery and development process,
http://www.novartis.com/innovation/research-development/drug-discovery-development-process/index.shtml

O'HEARE JAMES
Die Neuropsychologie des Hundes
Animal Learn Verlag 2009, p. 30-32

OLSON HARRY, BETTON GRAHAM, ROBINSON DENISE ET AL
Concordance of the Toxicity of Pharmaceuticals in Humans and in Animals
Regulatory Toxicology and Pharmacology 2000, Vol. 32, pp. 56-67

PHARMACEUTICAL RESEARCH AND DEVELOPMENT
Drug Discovery and Development,
http://www.innovation.org/drug_discovery/objects/pdf/RD_Brochure.pdf

RASHOTTE MICHAEL E., SMITH JAMES C., AUSTIN TRACEY, POLLITZ CELIA, CASTONGUAY THOMAS W., JONSSON LOGI
Twenty-Four-Hour Free-Feeding Patterns of Dogs Eating Dry Food,
Neuroscience & Biobehavioral Reviews 1984, Vol. 8, pp. 205-210

REILLY STEVE, BORNOVALOVA MARINA A.
Conditioned taste aversion and amygdala lesions in rat: A critical review
Neuroscience and Biobehavioral Reviews 2005, Vol. 29, pp. 1067-1088

ROHN CHRISTIANE
Man nennt mich Hundeflüsterin- Die Geheimnisse der Verständigung mit dem Tier; Editor ComArt, Weggis, 2007, 3rd edition, pp. 338-339

ROSS GR., GUSILS C., OLISZEWSKI R., DE HOLGADO SC, GONZÁLEZ SN.
Effects of probiotic administration in swine,
Journal of Bioscience and Bioengineering 2010, Vol. 109 (6), pp. 545-549

SAMBRAUS H.H., STEIGER A.
Grundbegriffe im Tierschutz
In: das Buch vom Tierschutz, Ferdinand Enke Verlag 1997, p. 33

SAMBRAUS H.H., STEIGER A.
Schmerz beim Tier
In: das Buch vom Tierschutz, Ferdinand Enke Verlag 1997, pp. 40-41

SANN H.
Notizeption und Schmerz
In: Physiologie der Haustiere, Editor von Engelhardt W., Enke Verlag Stuttgart 2000, pp. 76-77

SCHMIDT ROBERT F.
Thirst and Hunger: General Sensations
In: Fundamentals of Sensory Physiology, Springer Verlag 1977, New York, Heidelberg, Berlin, pp.8, 246-249

SCHMIDT ROBERT F.
Plastizität, Lernen, Gedächtnis
In: Physiologie des Menschen, Editor Schmidt Robert F. and Thews Gerhard, Springer-Verlag, 24. Auflage 1990, p. 164

SCHEMANN M.
Enterisches Nervensystem und Innervation des Magen-Darm-Traktes
In: Physiologie der Haustiere, Editor v. Engelhardt W., Enke Verlag Stuttgart 2000, pp. 309-317

SCHULZE V., ROEHE R., LORENZO BERMEJO J., LOOFT H. KALM E.
The influence of feeding behavior on feed intake curve parameters and performance traits of station-tested boars,
Livestock Production Science 2003, Vol. 82, pp. 105-116

SIMMONS R.D., KAISER F.C., PIERSON M.E., ROSAMOND J.R.
ARL 15849: a selective CCK-A agonist with anorectic activity in the rat and dog
Pharmacol. Biochem. Behavior, 1998, Vol. 59 (2), pp. 439-444

SMITH DAVID, TRENNERY PAUL
Non-rodent selection in pharmaceutical toxicology, a "points to consider" document
Association of the British Pharmaceutical Industry (ABPI) in conjunction with the UK Home Office, August 2002

SMITH DAVID, COMBES ROBERT, DEPELCHIN OLYMPE et al
Optimizing the design of preliminary toxicity studies for pharmaceutical safety testing in the dog
Regulatory Toxicology and Pharmacology 2005, Vol. 41, pp. 95-101

SWISS FEDERAL VETERINARY OFFICE
http://www.tv-statistik.bvet.admin.ch

VAN ZUTPHEN L.F.M., BAUMANS V., BEYNEN A.C.
Biology and husbandry of laboratory animals,
In "Principles of laboratory animal science", p. 47-50, Elsevier Verlag 1993

WEINGARTEN SALOMÉ, SENN MARKUS, LANGHANS WOLFGANG
Does a Learned Taste Aversion Contribute to the Anorectic Effect of Bacterial Lipopolysaccharide?
Physiology & Behavior 1993, Vol. 54, pp. 961-966

WINGFIELD JOHN C., RAMENOFSKY MARILYN
Hormones and the behavioral ecology of stress
In: Stress physiology in animals, Editor Balm Paul H., Sheffield Academic Press 1999, p. 4

ZORRILLA ERIC P., INOUE KOKI, FEKETE ÉVA M., TABARIN ANTOINE, VALDEZ GELNN R., KOOB GEORGE F.
Measuring meals: structure of prandial food and water intake of rats
American Journal of Physiol Regul integr Comp Physiol 2005, Vol. 288, pp. 1450-1467

8. Abbreviations

A

am: Ante meridium
AP: Area postrema
ATP: Adenosin triphosphat
AUC: Area under curve

B

BM: Body mass
Bvet: Bundesamt für Veterinärwesen

C

C: Celsius
CCK: Cholecystokinin
Cmax: maximum plasma concentration of the drug
CNS: Central nervous system
CS: Conditioned stimulus
CTA: Conditioned taste aversion
CSV: Comma-separated values
CVS: Cardiovascular system

D

DFI: Daily food intake

E

ECG: Electrocardiogram
EDTA: Ethylendiaminetetraacetic acid
e.g.: exempli gratia
EMA: European medicines agency
EMea: European agency for the evaluation of medicinal products
EnRep: Environmental Monitoring System
et al.: et alium

F

FDA: Food and drug administration

G

g: gram
GLP: Good laboratory practice
Dog ID: Dog Identification
GV-SOLAS: Gesellschaft für Versuchstierkunde

H

H: hours

I

ID: Identification

K

Kcal: kilocalorie
Kg: kilo gram

L

LASA: Laboratory animal science association
LPS: Lipopolysaccharides

M

M^2: Square meters
MDT: Meal duration time
ME: Metabolizable energy
Min: Minute
MJ: Megajoule
Ms: millisecond

N

NfE: Nitrogen free extract
NO: Nitric oxide
NPY: Neuropeptide Y
NTS: Solitari tract nucleus

P

pm: post meridium

S

S: seconds
SD: Standard deviation

T

Tmax: Time after administration of a drug when Cmax is reached
TNFα: Tumor necrosis factor alpha

U

US: Unconditioned stimulus
USA: United States of America

V

VIP: Vasoactive intestinal peptide
VpD: Visits per day

°: degree in Celsius
%: Percent

9. Appendix

Appendix 1: Food Consumption
Food composition of dog food 3353 from Provimi Kliba AG, Kaiseraugst
KLIBA NAFAG | PROVIMI KLIBA AG | CH-4303 Kaiseraugst | Tel. +41 61 816 16 16 | Fax +41 61 816 18 00 | kliba-nafag@provimi-kliba.ch | <u>www.kliba-nafag.ch</u>

Amino acids
Arginine 1.45 %
Lysine 1.23 %
Methionine 0.42 %
Methionine + cystine 0.85 %
Tryptophan 0.23 %
Threonine 0.82 %
Major Nutrients
Dry matter 88.0 %
Crude protein 22.5 %
Crude fat 6.0 %
Crude fiber 3.5 %
Crude ash 6.3 %
NFE 49.7 %
Gross energy 16.7 MJ/kg
Metabolisable energy 13.3 MJ/kg
Starch 33.0 %
Trace elements
Iron 200 mg/kg
Zinc 115 mg/kg
Copper 14 mg/kg
Iodine 1 mg/kg
Manganese 55 mg/kg
Selenium 0.25 mg/kg
Major mineral elements
Calcium 1.25 %
Phosphorus 0.90 %
Magnesium 0.20 %
Sodium 0.23 %
Potassium 0.67 %
Chlorine 0.34 %
Ingredients
Flacked cereals, wheat, poultry meal, flacked oats, soybean meal (NGMO), wheat middlings, soybean oil, wheat germ, corn (NGMO), minerals, vitamins, amino acids
Vitamins
Vitamin A 12'800 IU/kg
Vitamin D3 1'000 IU/kg
Vitamin E 130 mg/kg
Vitamin K3 5 mg/kg
Vitamin B1 23 mg/kg
Vitamin B2 13 mg/kg
Vitamin B6 9 mg/kg
Vitamin B12 0.05 mg/kg
Nicotinic acid 70 mg/kg

Pantothenic acid 30 mg/kg
Folic acid 2 mg/kg
Biotin 0.3 mg/kg
Choline 2'000 mg/kg
Vitamin C 370 mg/kg

Appendix 2: Tables of the various parameters to define the feeding behavior

Table 9.1 Average DFI of all females divided in their individual groups

DFI females (g) (mean values ± SD)	pretest	Main study	recovery
Group 1	270±39	284±51	310±63
Group 2	286±50	287±58	
Group 3	247±49	261±65	
Group 4	256±51	229±86	278±94
All groups	262±49	265±70	294±81
Total=Pt+MS+RC	265±65		

Table 9.2 Average MDT of all females divided in their individual groups

PT female (mins) (mean values ± SD)	pretest	Main study	recovery
Group 1	19.8±2.3	20.7±2	22.3±7.1
Group 2	20.3±2.1	22±1.9	
Group 3	18.7±2.1	20.4±2.1	
Group 4	17.1±3.4	17.4±5.9	24.1±10.4
All groups	19.7±4.5	20.1±5.9	23.2±8.6
Total=Pt+MS+RC	21.6±3.8		

Table 9.3 Average VpD of all females divided in their individual groups

VpD female (mean values ± SD)	pretest	Main study	recovery
Group 1	3.9±0.1	3.9±0.2	3.6±1.2
Group 2	4.2±0.2	3.9±0.2	
Group 3	3.8±0.2	3.6±0.2	
Group 4	3.7±0.2	3.3±0.3	3.9±1.2
All groups	3.9±0.9	3.7±1	3.8±1.2
Total=Pt+MS+RC	3.7±1.1		

Table 9.4 Average DFI of all males divided in their individual groups

DFI male (g) (mean values ± SD)	pretest	Main study	recovery
Group 1	335±41	350±49	373±70
Group 2	334±58	344±61	
Group 3	323±59	327±88	
Group 4	339±43	295±96	333±101
All groups	332±51	328±79	353±88
Total=Pt+MS+RC	329±73		

Table 9.5 Average MDT of all males divided in their individual groups

PT male (mins) (mean values ± SD)	pretest	Main study	recovery
Group 1	21.1±2.6	19.6±1.6	19.5±7
Group 2	22.4±4.2	19.6±3	
Group 3	18.6±2.9	17.8±1.8	
Group 4	16.7±3	19.4±6.2	19.1±9.9
All groups	18.6±4.1	18.3±5.6	19.3±7.9
Total=Pt+MS+RC	19±3.5		

Table 9.6 Average VpD of all males divided in their individual groups

VpD male (mean values ± SD)	pretest	Main study	recovery
Group 1	4.1±0.2	3.9±0.2	3.3±0.3
Group 2	4.1±0.2	3.9±0.3	
Group 3	4.1±0.2	3.6±0.4	
Group 4	3.9±0.2	3.4±0.2	3.5±0.3
All groups	4±1.1	3.7±1.2	3.4±1.4
Total=Pt+MS+RC	3.7±1.2		

Table 9.7 Average single meals of all females divided in their individual groups

Single meals female (g) (mean values ± SD)	pretest	Main study	recovery
Group 1	64±20	65±19	79±35
Group 2	61±22	64±26	
Group 3	63±25	65±24	
Group 4	62±22	61±24	66±22
All groups	62±22	64±23	72±30
Total=Pt+MS+RC	66±23		

Table 9.8 Average single meal duration of all females divided in their individual groups

Single PT female (mins) (mean values ± SD)	pretest	Main study	recovery
Group 1	5.1±1.3	5.1±1.2	5.7±2.1
Group 2	5±1.3	5.4±1.7	
Group 3	4.9±1.7	5.2±1.8	
Group 4	4.6±1.4	5.4±5.1	5.4±2.1
All groups	4.9±1.4	5.3±2.9	5.6±2.1
Total=Pt+MS+RC	5.1±1.9		

Table 9.9 Average single meals of all males divided in their individual groups

Single meals male (g) (mean values ± SD)	pretest	Main study	recovery
Group 1	73g±28	76g±30	91g±48
Group 2	70g±24	77g±28	
Group 3	77g±36	79g±36	
Group 4	78g±29	69g±33	84g±35
All groups	74g±30	75g±32	88g±43
Total=Pt+MS+RC	79g±30		

Table 9.10 Average single meal duration of all males divided in their individual groups

Single PT male (mins) (mean values ± SD)	pretest	Main study	recovery
Group 1	4.2±1.2	4.4±1.3	4.9±2.2
Group 2	4±1.3	4.3±1.4	
Group 3	4.1±1.2	4.3±1.4	
Group 4	4.6±1.5	4.3±2	5±1.8
All groups	4.2±1.3	4.3±1.6	5±2.1
Total=Pt+MS+RC	4.3±1.4		

Appendix 3 figures, charts and tables

Figure 2.1: Model of stress and distress 6

Figure 3.4: Process of drug development 12

Figure 4.1: Dog room from the front : *1= elevated platform, 2= privacy shield, 3= movable grid, 4= entrance to feeder* 17

Figure 4.2: Dog room from the side: *1= door opener* 18

Table 4.1: Recommended duration of repeated-dose toxicity studies (EMeA 2009) 19

Figure 4.3: Dogfeeder from the outside: *Black arrows point to the entrances of the feeder, 1= side protection, 2: silo* 23

Figure 4.4: Inside part of the Dogfeeder: *1= transponder receiver, 2= Balance, 3= Food bowl, 4= Food access door, 5= electropneumatic pistons* 23

Figure 4.5: Food bowl and transponder receiver: *1= Food bowl, 2= transponder receiver, 3= Food access door*......24

Figure 4.6: Implant: the black arrow points to the implant......24

Figure 4.7: Required points to get access to the food bowl......25

Figure 4.8: Display and control monitor......26

Figure 4.9: Selected study from the FeeditManager......27

Figure 4.10: Illustration of the different parameter used for the meal definition: *1= Intermeal interval*......28

Figure 4.11: Window with the defined parameters: *1= Intermeal Interval, 2= minimum intake, 3= minimal total single meal amount*......29

Figure 4.12: Summarized visits into the defined meal: *1= entry time into the feeder, 2= amount/time, 3= Meal sum: total of counted meals, 4= Sum: Total of the daily intake with residuals smaller than the minimal meal amount; 5= single meal duration time in sec.*......29

Figure 4.13: An error example: one meal measured four times......30

Chart 5.1: Box plot of the DFI of all females divided into the three study phases......32

Chart 5.2: Box plot of the DFI of all males divided into the three study phases......32

Table 5.1: Mean values of food intake of the females of all studies divided into the three study phases......34

Table 5.2: Mean values of food intake of the males of all studies divided into the three study phases......34

Chart 5.3: Average of DFI of all females divided into the four dose groups......35

Chart 5.4: Average of DFI of males divided into the four dose groups......36

Chart 5.5: Average of the daily MDT of all females divided into the four dose groups......37

Chart 5.6: Average of the daily MDT of all males divided into the four dose groups......37

Table 5.3: Mean values of all females in group 4 divided into the three study phases......38

Table 5.4: Mean values of all males in group 4 divided into the three study phases......38

Chart 5.7: Average of DFI of females of study A......40

Chart 5.8: Average of DFI of female group 4......41

Chart 5.9: Average of DFI of males of study A......42

Chart 5.10: DFI and VpD of one dog out of male group 1......43

Chart 5.11: Average of DFI of female group 1,3,and 4......44

Chart 5.12: Average of DFI of female group 4 of study B......45

Chart 5.13: Average of the single meals of one dog of female group 4 of study B, divided into the timeslots......46

Chart 5.14: Average of the single meals of the same dog as in chart 5.13, only the early phase; * = the break between day 0 and day 6 with no food intake 47

Chart 5.15: Average daily food intake of male group 1-4 from the example study 48

Chart 5.16: DFI during pretest and main phase of the two dogs of male group 4 48

Chart 5.17: DFI during the recovery phase of the two dogs of male group 4 49

Chart 5.18: Average DFI of female group 4 of study C 50

Chart 5.19: Average DFI of male group 4 of study C 51

Chart 5.20: Average DFI and VpD of one female of group 4 of study C 52

Chart 5.21: DFI and MDT of one male dog of high dose group 4 52

Chart 5.22: Average DFI of female group 2 53

Table 5.5: Symptoms of two female dogs of the low dose group (Group 2) 54

Chart 5.23: Average DFI of male group 2 55

Table 5.6: Symptoms of two animals of the male group 2 55

Chart 5.24: Average daily food intake compared between group 1 and 4 of both sexes 56

Table 5.7: Symptoms of one male dog of high dose group 4 57

Table 5.8: Symptoms of a male dog of high dose 4 57

Chart 5.25: Average of DFI of female group 4 in pretest, main phase and recovery; (error bars with 5%) 58

Chart 5.26: Average DFI of female group 1-4 of the example study 59

Chart 5.27: Mean values of DFI of all five animals (1-5) of female group 4, divided into pretest, main phase and recovery; (error bars with 5%) 59

Chart 5.28: Average total food intake of all four male dogs (1-4) of group 4, divided into pretest, main phase and recovery; (errors bars with 5%) 60

Chart 5.29: Mean values of MDT of male group 4 (1-4), divided into pretest, main phase and recovery; (error bars with 5%) 61

Chart 5.30: Mean values of DFI of male group 1 (1-5), divided into pretest, main phase and recovery; (error bars with 5%) 62

Chart 5.31: Mean values of MDT of male group 1 (1-5), divided into pretest, main phase and recovery (error bars with 5%) 62

Table 5.9: symptoms of one male dog of high dose group 4 63

Table 5.10: Symptoms of one female dog of high dose group 4 63

Chart 5.32: DFI and total visits of one dog for all three study phases; pretest, main phase and recovery: *Black arrow=start of the main phase; violet arrow=start of the recovery phase* 64

Chart 5.33: DFI and total visits of one dog for all three study phases; pretest, main phase and recovery: *Black arrow=start of the main phase; violet arrow=start of the recovery phase* 65

Chart 5.34: Appearance of the different symptoms in percentage: *1= salivation, 2= vomiting, 3= diarrhea, 4= limbs, 5= neurolog. signs, 6= behavioral signs,7= posture, 8= respiration; the percentage is referred to the total number of animals with or without symptoms* 67

Table 6.1: Number of animals used in experiments 2009 (Swiss federal veterinary office)... 68

Table 6.2: Number of animals used in experiments 2008 (Swiss federal veterinary office)... 68

10. Acknowledgement

My special thanks go to Professor Dr. Thomas Lutz of the Institute of Veterinary Physiology at the Vetsuisse Faculty in Zürich and Dr. Rudolf Pfister, head of animal husbandry in Toxicology, Novartis Pharma Basel for their great support and helpful inputs when I needed them. I'm also very grateful for the quick reviews of my drafts.

I also want to thank Professor Dr. Paul Torgerson for introducing me into the sophistically world of statistics, answering all my statistical questions and for taking on the role of co-referee.

Many thanks go to Christian Waldmann, who developed the software of the Feeding system for me. He spent a lot of time to add new functions into the software to simplify the analysis of the whole data.

I would like to mention Ionel Onofrescu who helped me to improve my skills in excel and helping me with the pivot-table. I'm very grateful for his help. I also thank Ian Bunn for taking the time to review my dissertation. He has done it in such a short period.

Warmly thanks go to Tom Wernli and the non-rodent team who took their time to answer my many questions about the dog feeding system and for giving me a great time in Novartis.

And last but not least, I want to thank the whole team of the toxicology of Novartis Pharma Basel and all others, who supported me in any way. Thank you!

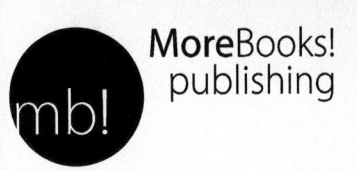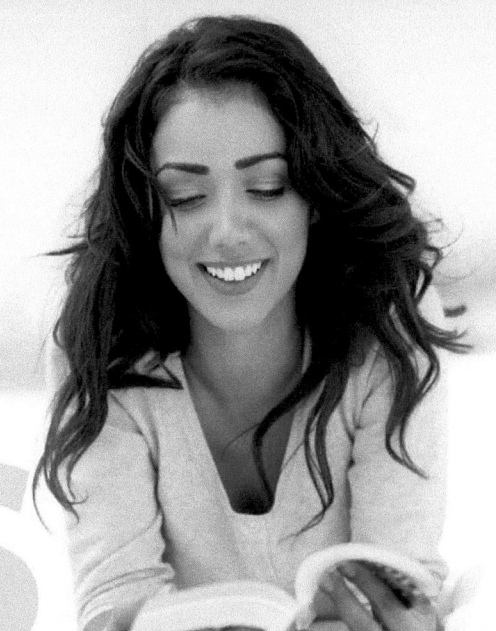

i want morebooks!

Buy your books fast and straightforward online - at one of world's fastest growing online book stores! Environmentally sound due to Print-on-Demand technologies.

Buy your books online at

www.get-morebooks.com

Kaufen Sie Ihre Bücher schnell und unkompliziert online – auf einer der am schnellsten wachsenden Buchhandelsplattformen weltweit! Dank Print-On-Demand umwelt- und ressourcenschonend produziert.

Bücher schneller online kaufen

www.morebooks.de

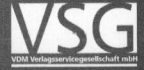 VDM Verlagsservicegesellschaft mbH
Heinrich-Böcking-Str. 6-8   Telefon: +49 681 3720 174   info@vdm-vsg.de
D - 66121 Saarbrücken   Telefax: +49 681 3720 1749   www.vdm-vsg.de

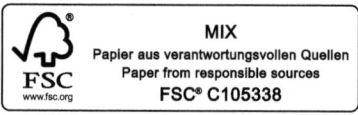

Printed by Books on Demand GmbH, Norderstedt / Germany